★ THE COMPLETE ★

DIABETES

COOKBOOK

FOR BEGINNERS

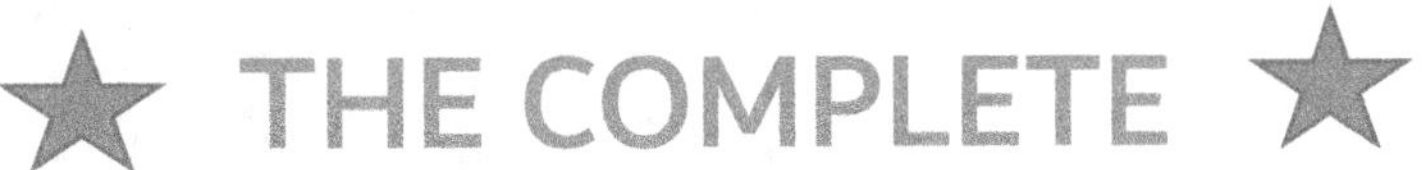

Simple and Delicious Recipe to Manage Your Diabetes with 2000+ Days of Low-Sugar and Low-Carb Recipes, accompanied by A **30-DAY MEAL PLAN** Designed to Establish Healthy Eating Habits

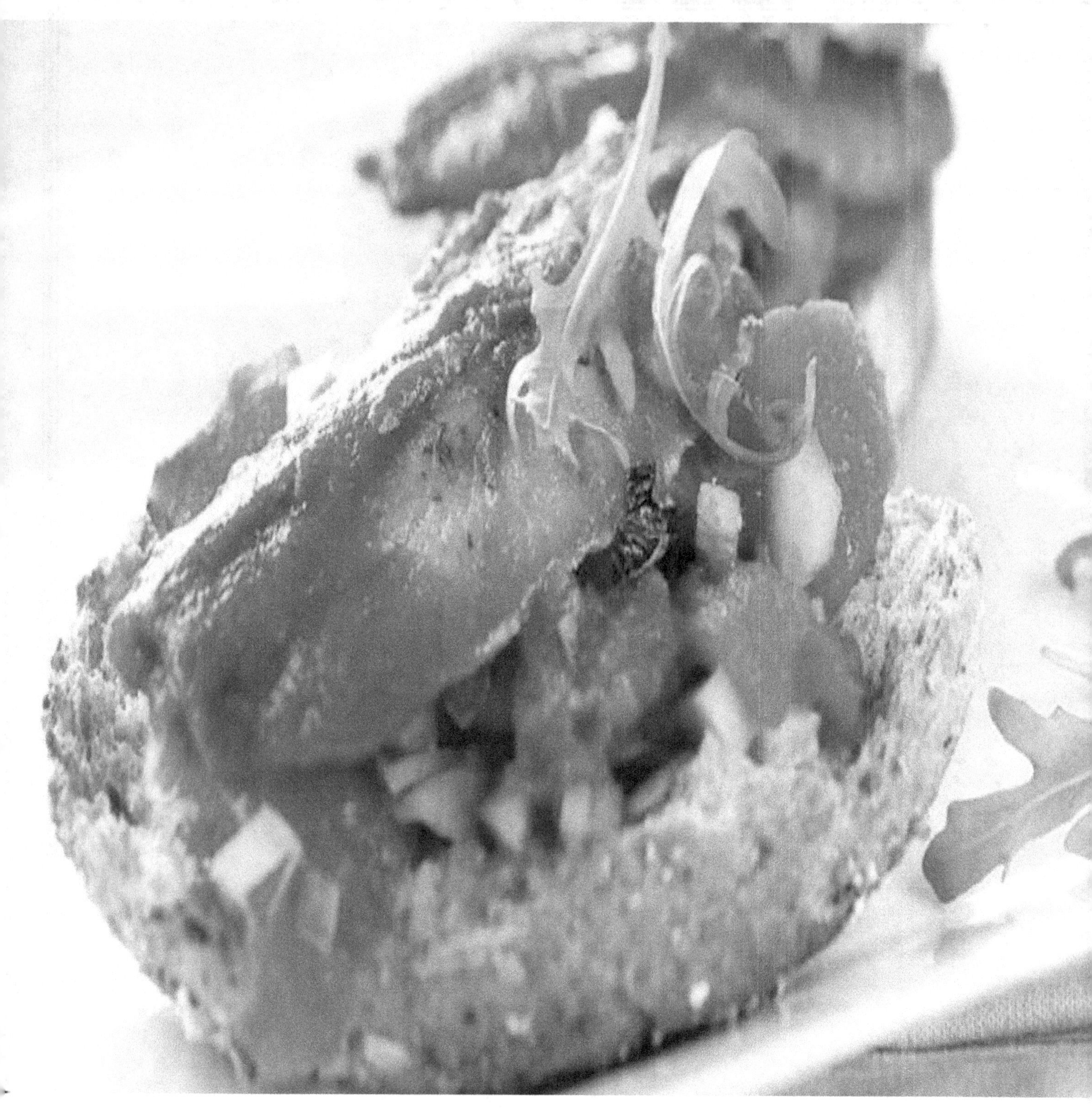

PAULA J. EVANS

30-DAYS MEAL PLAN

Day	Breakfast	Lunch	Dinner	Snacks	Dessert
1	Greek Yogurt and Berries Parfait	Grilled Chicken Salad	Baked Salmon with Asparagus	Cucumber and Hummus Slices	Chia Pudding with Berries
2	Oatmeal with Almonds and Blueberries	Quinoa Salad with Veggies	Lemon Pepper Shrimp in Air Fryer	Baked Zucchini Chips	Fresh Fruit Salad with Mint Yogurt
3	Scrambled Eggs with Spinach	Cauliflower Mashed Potatoes	Ginger Sesame Salmon	Apple and Peanut Butter Slices	Dark Chocolate-Dipped Strawberries
4	Avocado Toast with Poached Eggs	Red Beans and Rice	Tuna Sweetcorn Casserole	Veggie Sticks with Hummus	Greek Yogurt with Honey and Nuts
5	Banana Walnut Pancakes	Balsamic Cabbage	Swordfish Steak	Cottage Cheese and Pineapple Delight	Fresh Berries with Whipped Cream
6	Sunflower Seeds Dressing Salad	Black Bean and Vegetable Burrito	Tarragon Cod Fillets	Apple and Peanut Butter Slices	Dark Chocolate-Dipped Strawberries
7	Chia Pudding with Berries	Roasted Tomato Brussels Sprouts	Sesame Shrimp Mix	Cottage Cheese and Sliced Peaches	Fruit Salad with Mint Yogurt
8	Greek Yogurt and Berries Parfait	Tofu with Brussels Sprouts	Lemon Salmon with Kaffir Lime	Veggie Sticks with Hummus	Fresh Berries with Whipped Cream
9	Oatmeal with Almonds and Blueberries	Chili Broccoli	Baked Fish Served with Vegetables	Cucumber and Hummus Slices	Chia Pudding with Berries
10	Scrambled Eggs with Spinach	Paprika Brussels Sprouts	Tuna Sweetcorn Casserole	Baked Zucchini Chips	Greek Yogurt with Honey and Nuts

11	Avocado Toast with Poached Eggs	Red Cabbage Salad	Sesame Shrimp Mix	Apple and Peanut Butter Slices	Dark Chocolate-Dipped Strawberries
12	Banana Walnut Pancakes	Green Beans with Paprika	Spicy Cod	Veggie Sticks with Hummus	Fresh Fruit Salad with Mint Yogurt
13	Sunflower Seeds Dressing Salad	Chili Broccoli	Swordfish Steak	Cottage Cheese and Pineapple Delight	Fruit Salad with Mint Yogurt
14	Greek Yogurt and Berries Parfait	Paprika Brussels Sprouts	Tarragon Cod Fillets	Cucumber and Hummus Slices	Chia Pudding with Berries
15	Oatmeal with Almonds and Blueberries	Green Beans in Oven	Ginger Sesame Salmon	Apple and Peanut Butter Slices	Dark Chocolate-Dipped Strawberries
16	Scrambled Eggs with Spinach	Rosemary Potatoes	Lemon Pepper Shrimp in Air Fryer	Veggie Sticks with Hummus	Fresh Berries with Whipped Cream
17	Avocado Toast with Poached Eggs	Paprika Brussels Sprouts	Swordfish Steak	Cottage Cheese and Sliced Peaches	Fresh Fruit Salad with Mint Yogurt
18	Banana Walnut Pancakes	Mashed Pumpkin	Tarragon Cod Fillets	Baked Zucchini Chips	Greek Yogurt with Honey and Nuts
19	Sunflower Seeds Dressing Salad	Chili Broccoli	Lemon Salmon with Kaffir Lime	Apple and Peanut Butter Slices	Dark Chocolate-Dipped Strawberries
20	Greek Yogurt and Berries Parfait	Green Beans in Oven	Sesame Shrimp Mix	Veggie Sticks with Hummus	Chia Pudding with Berries
21	Oatmeal with Almonds and Blueberries	Mashed Pumpkin	Baked Fish Served with Vegetables	Cottage Cheese and Pineapple Delight	Fruit Salad with Mint Yogurt

22	Scrambled Eggs with Spinach	Rosemary Potatoes	Spicy Cod	Cucumber and Hummus Slices	Fresh Berries with Whipped Cream
23	Avocado Toast with Poached Eggs	Green Beans with Paprika	Lemon Pepper Shrimp in Air Fryer	Apple and Peanut Butter Slices	Dark Chocolate-Dipped Strawberries
24	Banana Walnut Pancakes	Mashed Pumpkin	Tuna Sweetcorn Casserole	Veggie Sticks with Hummus	Greek Yogurt with Honey and Nuts
25	Sunflower Seeds Dressing Salad	Chili Broccoli	Swordfish Steak	Cottage Cheese and Sliced Peaches	Fresh Fruit Salad with Mint Yogurt
26	Greek Yogurt and Berries Parfait	Green Beans in Oven	Tarragon Cod Fillets	Baked Zucchini Chips	Chia Pudding with Berries
27	Oatmeal with Almonds and Blueberries	Mashed Pumpkin	Ginger Sesame Salmon	Apple and Peanut Butter Slices	Dark Chocolate-Dipped Strawberries
28	Scrambled Eggs with Spinach	Rosemary Potatoes	Lemon Salmon with Kaffir Lime	Veggie Sticks with Hummus	Fruit Salad with Mint Yogurt
29	Avocado Toast with Poached Eggs	Green Beans with Paprika	Spicy Cod	Cottage Cheese and Pineapple Delight	Greek Yogurt with Honey and Nuts
30	Banana Walnut Pancakes	Mashed Pumpkin	Baked Fish Served with Vegetables	Cucumber and Hummus Slices	Fresh Berries with Whipped Cream

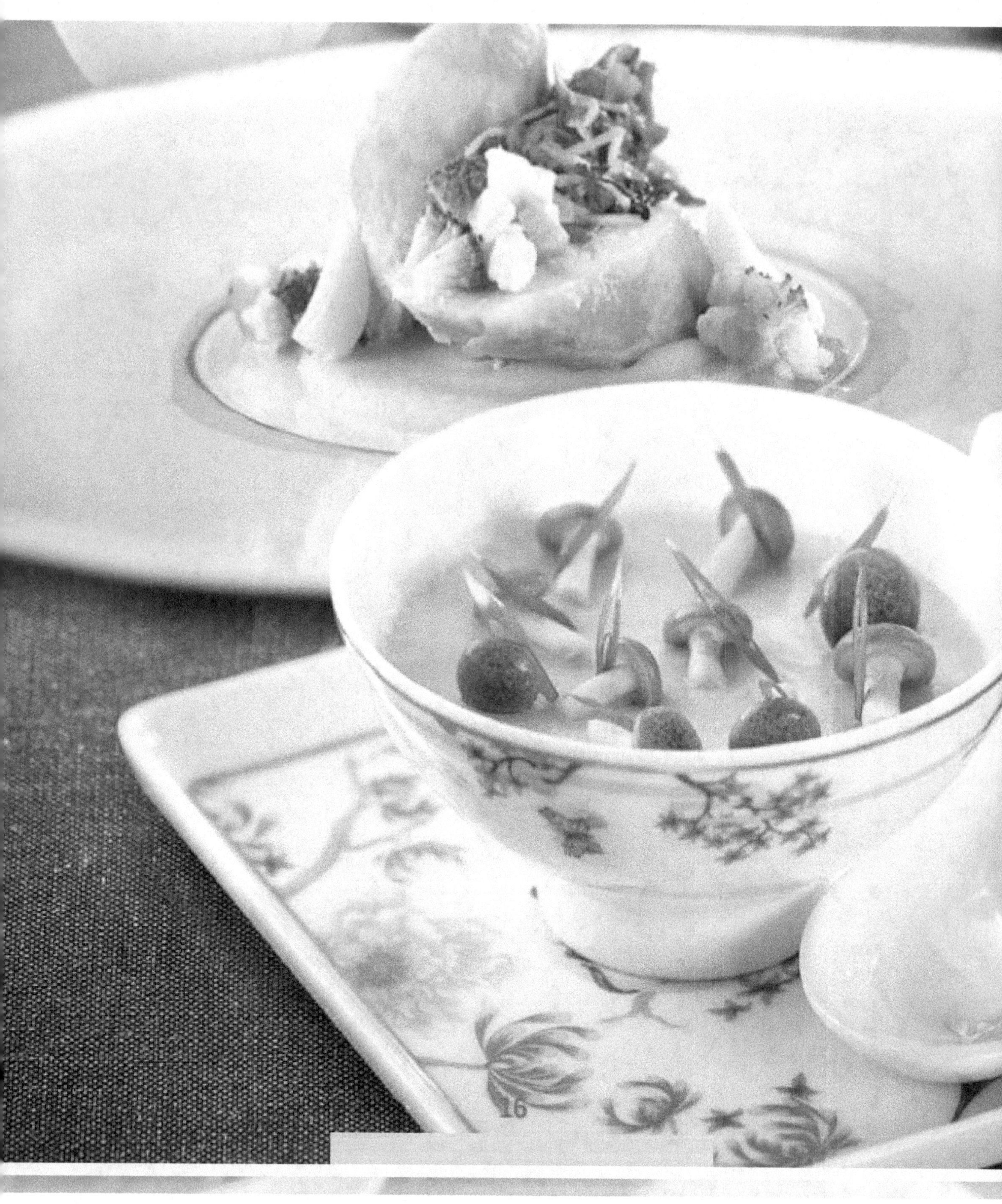

Copyright © 2023, Paula J Evans.

All rights reserved.

For permission requests, please contact the author

Disclaimer:

The information contained in this book is provided for educational and informational purposes only. It is not intended as a substitute for professional advice, diagnosis, or treatment. Always seek the advice of your physician, therapist, or other qualified healthcare provider with any questions you may have regarding a medical condition or treatment.

The author and publisher of this book have made every effort to ensure the accuracy of the information presented. However, they make no representations or warranties of any kind, express or implied, about the completeness, accuracy, reliability, suitability, or availability with respect to the information, products, services, or related graphics contained in this book for any purpose.

Supper Foods for Diabetes

NUTRITIONAL BENEFITS

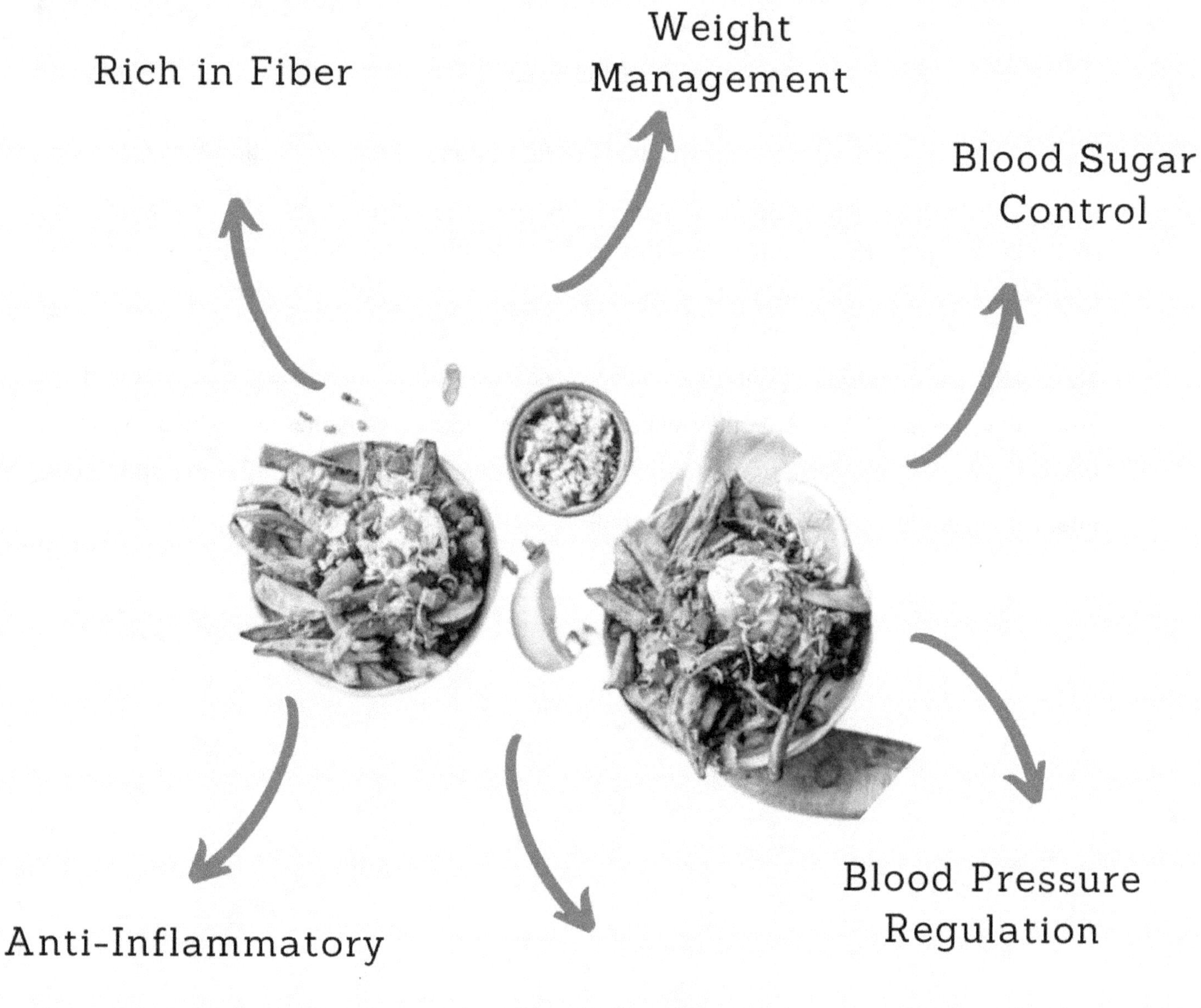

TABLE OF CONTENTS

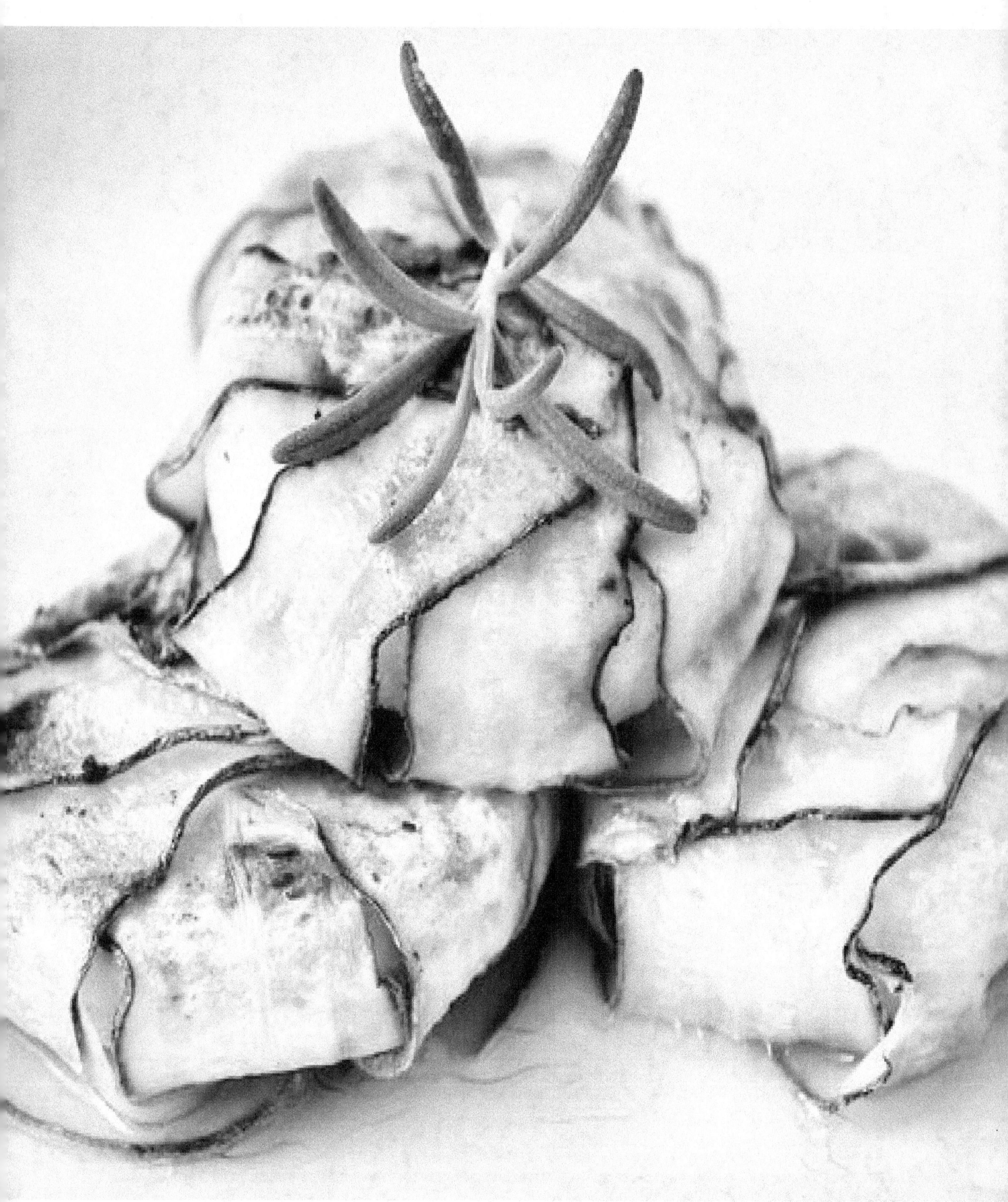

INTRODUCTION

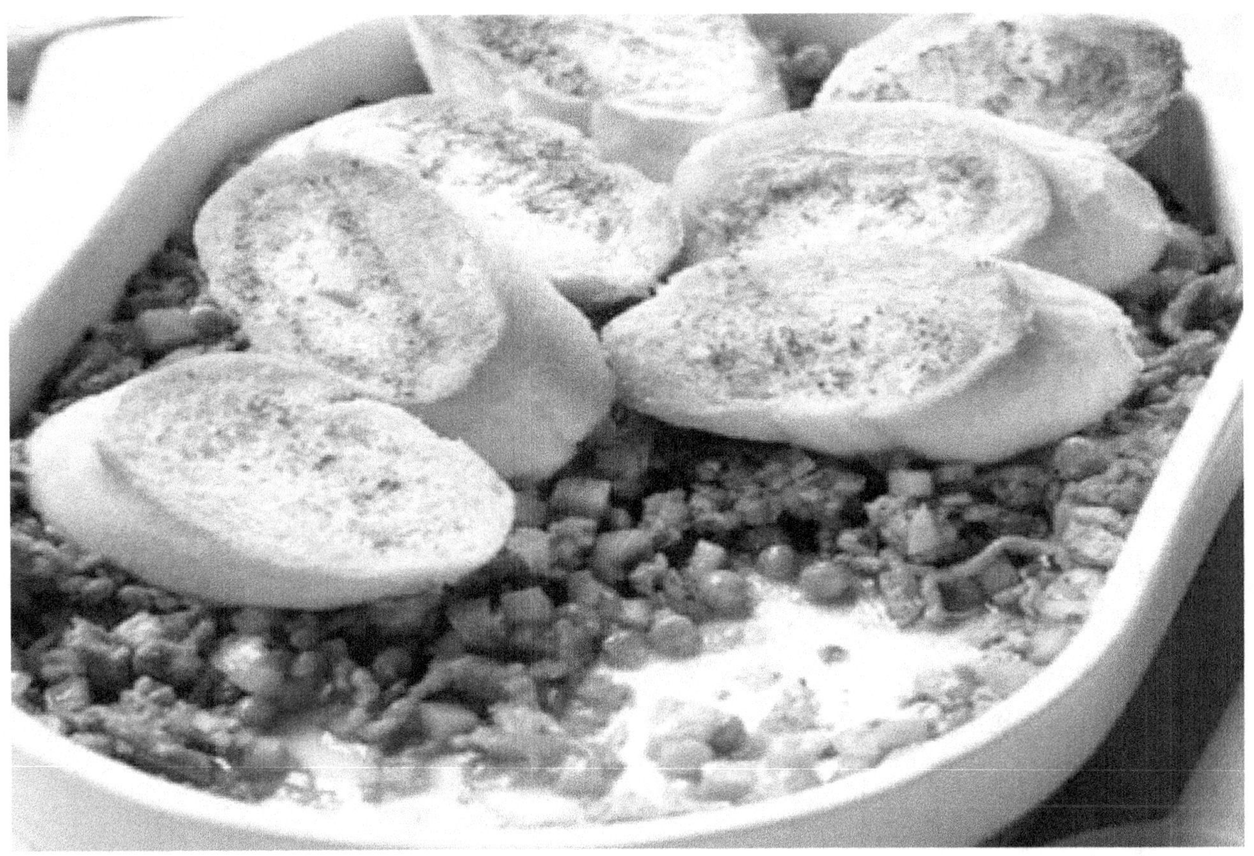

In America, every 17 seconds a new patient is diagnosed with diabetes.

This is why, to today, more than 37.3 million US residents suffer from the condition.

But that's hardly the most troubling statistic.

In fact, just at this now, 1 in 3 Americans is at danger of acquiring the disease but is unaware of it.

And consequently, they don't even realize the risks that the illness exposes them to.

For example, a 94% increased probability of developing certain forms of cancer

– compared to a healthy individual.

Perhaps this is also why the "silent killer" – as some physicians call diabetes – claimed more than 1.5 million lives in 2019 alone.

It may seem startling, but regrettably, it's the terrible truth.

So, if you or a family have just been diagnosed with diabetes, you may feel confused and concerned.

You may be wondering what hazards you face and what your life will be like from now on.

If you need to give up your favorite foods and stick to a dull diet.

If that is the case, I have wonderful news for you.

In fact, today I will answer all these questions so that I may make things clearer for you.

To start with, I'll explain the difference between prediabetes and type 2 diabetes.

I will also show you the one reason that puts you at danger of having the disease…

… and routines to avoid, regulate, or even reverse it.

Finally, I will reveal the dietary strategies, the foods to keep away from, and those that will help you manage diabetes.

All that without boring diets, giving up tasty foods, or working your guts off in the gym.

In fact, in this recipe book, you will find tons of scrumptious dishes to assist you manage the condition.

Therefore, you may sit down at the dinner table and have 3 or 4 great meals every day.

Lunch and supper, day after day.

As a result, eating will become a real joy and you will not even feel like you are "dieting".

Then, are you ready to find out how to control your diabetes, avoid it, or even reverse it?

Great, let's get started!

What is Diabetes?

The difference between Prediabetes and Type 2 Diabetes

In this first introduction, I'll show you the difference between the two situations.

But let me simply explain what it is all about — and why these troubles occur.

Diabetes and prediabetes occur when your blood sugar is too high — in other words, when you have too much sugar in your blood.

This occurs for a simple reason: insulin resistance.

But what is it?

Let me clarify.

Your pancreas generates a hormone called insulin, whose aim is to control blood sugar.

To achieve this, it permits glucose to enter the cells, so that they dispose of it by utilizing it as an energy source.

When your body fails to utilize its insulin well – or does not create enough of it – your sugars will become caught outside your cells and stagnate in your bloodstream.

This is how your blood sugar increases and insulin resistance develops.

The reasons why this occurs are many, and I will expose them soon.

Now that I've showed you how prediabetes and diabetes develop, I'll explain the

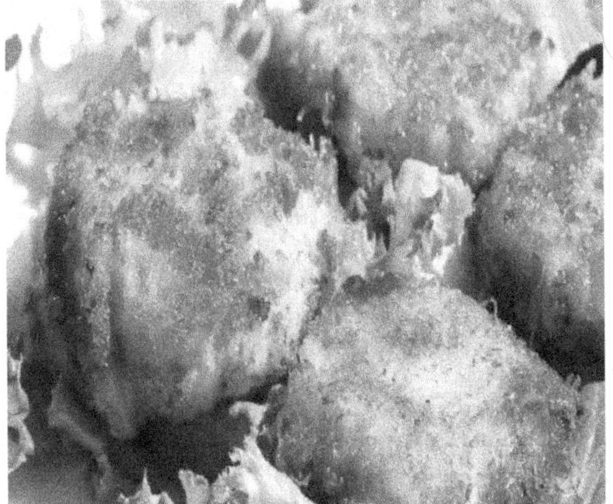

differences between the two conditions.

As I have previously mentioned, the two diseases are distinct.

Prediabetes. This is the early stage of the issue — a type of "wake-up call," so to speak.

Insulin does not execute its duty as it should and the blood sugar level begins to rise.

We talk about prediabetes in two circumstances: when fasting blood glucose is between 100 and 125 mg/dl; when blood glucose after meals is between 140 and 199 mg/dl.

Often, this syndrome progresses into type 2 diabetes. However, if you are familiar with the correct ways to curb the issue, you can make it regress and vanish. So, in a little while, I'll teach you how to counteract this problem.

The disease is typically the development of prediabetes. In this instance, insulin performs its role in an increasingly unsatisfactory manner.

We talk about type 2 diabetes in the following cases: when fasting blood glucose is > 126 mg/dl; when blood glucose after meals is > 200 mg/dl.

Sometimes, in this case, you may also need to take drugs to balance your blood sugar.

However, I have some wonderful news for you.

Prediabetes and type 2 diabetes can actually be avoided, managed, or even reversed.

To accomplish so, you need to work on a single very important factor: insulin resistance.

If you can tackle insulin resistance and teach your body how to effectively handle this hormone, then you may be able to say goodbye to diabetes.

So, today I want to teach you precisely what you need to do to take care of your body, contain the problem of high blood sugar, and go back to living a regular life.

But first, let me show you what are the factors that put you – or maybe a loved one – at risk of having diabetes or failing to manage it.

2. The 6 primary reasons – and why you need to know them straight from the start

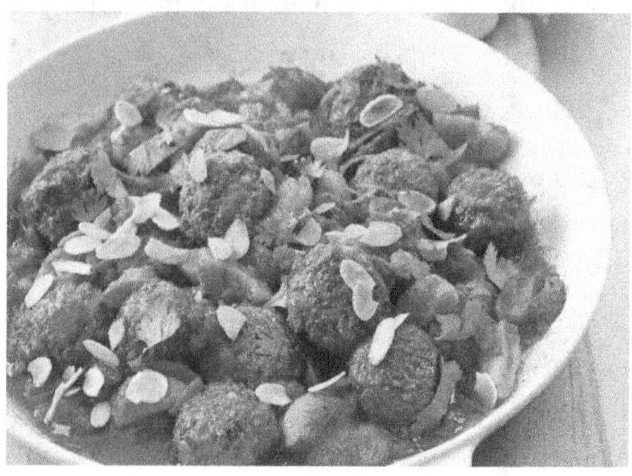

Now, I want to inform you what unhealthy habits enhance your chances of suffering from diabetes and prediabetes.

As I told you earlier, the condition often starts growing with insulin resistance.

So, these are the circumstances that put you at risk.

- Prediabetes. This is the key because that raises your chances of developing diabetes. Based on the latest study, more than 96 million Americans are now in this situation. It is precisely when you find yourself at this point, that you should do everything you can to arrest the progression of the illness in time.

Therefore, first and foremost, pay attention if you or your loved ones are experiencing symptoms such as:

- frequent urination;
- increased thirst;
- fatigue;
- blurred vision;
- tingling in your hands and feet;
- sudden weight loss;
- constant hunger.

These are some of the "Red flags" of prediabetes — and also of type 2 diabetes.

So, in the following chapter, I'll show you the tactics and habits to get the situation back on track before it degenerates. Excessive weight.

Obesity and being overweight are two conditions that exacerbate your insulin resistance worse, putting you at risk for prediabetes and ultimately type 2 diabetes. Just consider that nowadays, about 70% of the American population is overweight – which is exactly why it is a significant cause of diabetes.

Sedentary lifestyle. According to the latest study, sedentary persons are twice as likely to acquire prediabetes or diabetes, compared to those who exercise frequently. Additionally, being sedentary raises the probability of death from cardiovascular disease by 90%. Hypertension. High blood pressure is typically associated to the development of diabetes and prediabetes. In fact, according to the American Diabetes Association, 2 out of 3 patients with diabetes also suffer from hypertension.

- These two disorders may feed one other and make each other worse. Therefore, the following chapter will disclose several routines to reduce your blood pressure. Age. Research shows that the risk of acquiring diabetes increases beyond 45 years of age. But the scenario gets much further after you approach 65 years. In fact, according to the newest data, in this age range, at least 3 out of 4 people have prediabetes or diabetes – and regrettably, many of them are still ignorant of it. So, particularly as you become older, you should keep an eye on your blood sugar and lifestyle.

Genetics. This is the single aspect you can't genuinely control. Type 1 diabetes is a disorder that commonly runs in the family via genes. Therefore, if someone in your family has this condition, you should be much more alert to all the things you can control.

These are the primary reasons why you develop insulin resistance — and as a consequence, prediabetes or diabetes.

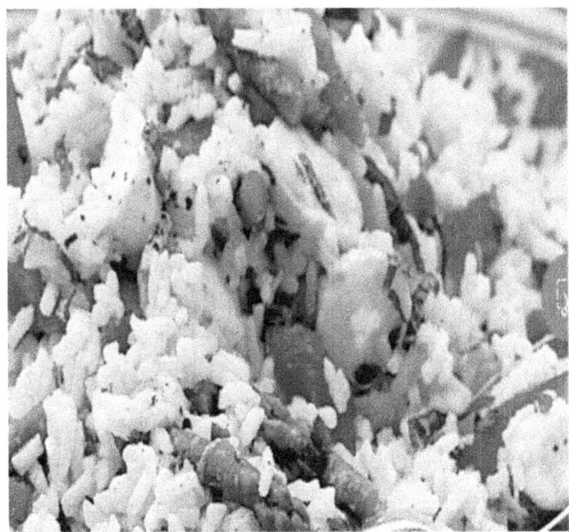

Now, you need to realize that tackling these issues as soon as possible can make a tremendous impact in your life – or those of your loved ones.

In reality, persons with diabetes incur several risks associated to their condition, as I told you at the beginning of this section.

For example, 230 diabetic individuals in America are amputated every day because of their illness.

But that's not all.

According to Cleveland Clinic, if you have diabetes, you have a 50% increased chance of having a stroke.

You see, this illness continuously puts your life (or that of your loved one) at danger.

That's why, in the following chapter, I'm going to divulge the practices that won't only help you manage diabetes, but enhance your overall health and minimize the risk of various ailments, including heart disease.

3. 8 behaviors that help you prevent, control and reverse the condition

As I told you, several healthy practices can help you battle diabetes.

Moreover, these recommendations will also help you improve your overall health.

This will minimize the danger of developing other ailments, as well as making you feel more active.

So, here are the 8 healthy behaviors you should adopt to avoid, treat or reverse diabetes.

1. Check your blood sugar level. Altered blood sugar is one of the earliest red flags for prediabetes and diabetes.

That's why you should monitor it.

Therefore, bear in mind that normal blood sugar levels are: between 70 and 99 mg/dl fasting; <140 mg/dl 2 hours after eating.

2. Check your blood pressure. As I mentioned before, hypertension is one of the primary causes of diabetes, therefore you should keep it under control. In fact, according to research issued by the cardiac Foundation, persons with diabetes have a 4-fold greater risk of having cardiac issues. As a result, you should periodically monitor your blood pressure. Remember that the ideal readings are less than 120/80 mmHg.

3. Exercise. Earlier, we observed that a sedentary lifestyle raises the risk not just of getting diabetes but also of cardiovascular illnesses.

That's why the National Institute of Diabetes and Digestive and Kidney Diseases suggests at least 30 minutes of exercise, 5 times a week. No need to undertake hard and exhausting workouts. To start with, even a stroll is fine.

Get adequate sleep. A mature person should sleep 7-8 hours a night. In fact, a research published in the National Library of Medicine (PubMed), shows how inadequate slumber may modify the amount of glucose in the blood. Quit smoking. I don't even need to tell you: smoking is incredibly hazardous and increases the chance of major issues like cancer. It also harms the airways and heart. Lose weight. I mentioned earlier that obesity and overweight are among the leading causes of prediabetes and diabetes. That's why you should aim to enhance your fitness levels. There's no need to strive to lose too much weight all at once.

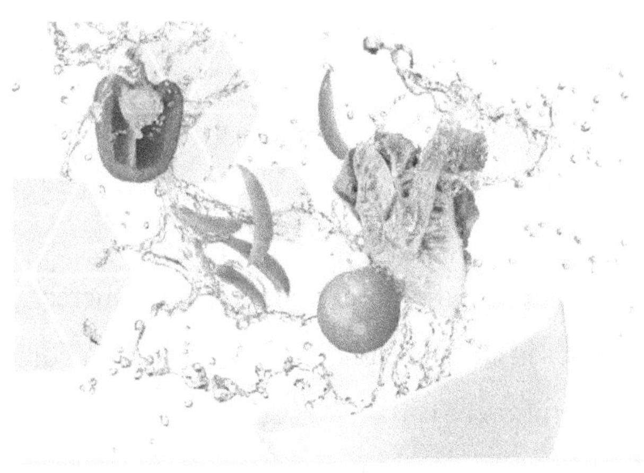

To begin with, the National Institute of Diabetes and Digestive and Kidney Diseases suggests decreasing between 5% and 7% of your weight. For instance, if you weigh 200 lbs., then your initial goal should be to shed between 10 and 14 lbs. Manage stress. A 2020 study shows the association between stress and type 2 diabetes. Indeed, when you are stressed your body boosts the production of chemicals such as cortisol.

This produces an imbalance in blood sugar.

Therefore, you should strive to minimize your stress levels, possibly by taking up activities such as yoga or meditation.

Exercise might also help.

Follow a proper diet. This is possibly the single most crucial part of preventing diabetes, managing it, or reversing it. This is why I chose to devote the following chapter to eating strategies that might aid you in this task.

Now, let's get into the meat of this section and look together at how you should adjust your diet.

4. Diabetes diet: 8+1 stages for optimal structure

I want to explain the nutritional ways to control your prediabetes or type 2 diabetes.

I chose to arrange my advice in 8+1 different parts, in order to make each aspect clearer.

Now I'm going to teach you precisely how to set up a healthy diet.

1. Carbohydrates

When addressing diabetes, we immediately think of carbs.

Most individuals feel they will have to remove them totally from their diet and give up permanently a plate of spaghetti, a slice of pizza, or a delectable bread roll.

The fact is completely different.

Obviously, you need to manage your intake and abstain from overindulging.

However, you may still incorporate them in your diet.

An excellent technique may be to eat them at the end of your meal, possibly starting with a bowl of veggies.

Besides improving your sensation of satiety, they will assist you slow down the assimilation of carbs.

Thus, you can avoid rapid glycemic spikes.

2. Glycemic index

Another essential aspect: not all carbohydrates are created equal.

Indeed, they vary dependent on their glycemic index.

Are you wondering what it means?

It is the pace at which a given food increases blood sugar levels, and it is rated with a number ranging from 0 to 100.

Foods come into 3 categories

Low glycemic index: between 0 and 55; Medium glycemic index: between 56 and 69; High glycemic index: between 70 and 100.

Please notice!

The cooking process impacts the glycemic index. For example, pasta cooked al dente has a lower index than overcooked pasta. Therefore, choose for light cooking and raw meals.

In your diet, you should thus favor foods with a low or medium glycemic index – but also be cautious about which cooking techniques you employ. In the next two chapters, I will tell you precisely which foods to pick — and which to avoid.

3. Fiber

As I indicated before, fiber helps you increase your sensation of fullness and slow down your absorption of carbs.

For this reason, each of your meals should contain veggies and fruit. Be aware, though!

Fruit includes sugars, therefore you should consume it in moderation.

Above all, not all fruits are the same.

That's why I'll show you the ones you should prefer.

4. Portions.

Many individuals feel they need to maintain a count of every single calorie they intake.

Of course, you have to be conscious of how much you consume; but typically you won't need to be particularly exact.

So, to minimize unneeded tension, you can try the following technique.

Picture splitting the dish in half.

In one half, you will arrange your veggies.

Now, further split the remaining half in two.

One quarter will be carbs, the other proteins.

That's how you make a balanced dish, without weighing every single ingredient.

Remember the "Health dish" (25% carbs from cereals, 25% proteins and 50% carbs from vegetables).

5. Calories

Adjusting the calories, you consume is important to keep your diabetes under control.

As I told you previously, you don't need to track them with extraordinary precision.

However, it is all-important that you should avoid being on a high-calorie regimen regularly.

If you question what this implies, simply know that it is the condition in which your calorie intake is larger than your calorie consumption.

Indeed, research reveals how a hyper caloric diet develops insulin resistance.

That's why you should try to just eat what your body demands.

6. Water You should consume between 1.5 and 2 liters of water a day.

However, this differs from person to person.

Besides keeping you hydrated and healthy, several new research published in the National Library of Medicine demonstrate that proper hydration may reduce your blood sugar levels.

7. Probiotics

They are "good bacteria" with a variety of beneficial impacts on the body.

Some new research, also published in the National Library of Medicine, reveal how they may help to managing blood sugar levels.

In the penultimate chapter, I will show you some of the foods high in probiotics that you should include in your diet.

8. Fats

Many people are not aware of this, but fats might really be more detrimental than sugars for diabetes.

Again: not ALL fats, certainly.

As a matter of fact, there are excellent ones and poor ones.

The latter — that is, saturated fats – are the ones you should reduce.

They may elevate your cholesterol levels and expose you to the danger of cardiovascular disease – which will be high to start with if you suffer from diabetes.

The final advice I want to share with you is that you should check the food labels when you go shopping.

In reality, many meals that you might consider "healthy" … … really include hidden carbohydrates and fats.

So, before placing a product in your shopping basket, read the label and check the following entries:

sugar; saturated fats.

There is no specific value, but the lower the better.

Now that I have showed you the dietary strategies to avoid prediabetes or diabetes, moderate, or cure it… … you're finally ready to find out what foods you should stay away from.

5. The list of items you should avoid

In this chapter, I want to provide you a list of foods that are dangerous to your health – if you have diabetes.

Needless to say, this does not imply that you will have to exclude these foods from your diet permanently.

However, depending on the severity of your condition, you will need to reduce their consumption.

I have chosen to organize the foods by category, in order to offer you a better understanding.

1. Carbohydrates

- Any having a high glycemic index.
- White rice
- Pasta
- White bread
- French fries and chips
- Savory crackers
- Corn flakes
- Puffed rice
- Popcorn Pizza
- Rice cakes

2. Protein in general, any fat and processed meats.

- Bacon
- Fried meat
- Fried fish
- Sausages
- Fatty beef burgers
- Processed meats
- Chicken with skin

3. Vegetables

- Reduce your consumption of starchy veggies.
- Cooked carrots
- Potatoes
- Canned vegetables
- Vegetables sautéed with oil or butter
- Beetroot Pumpkin

- Bananas
- Watermelon
- Dried fruit
- Canned fruit in syrup
- Fruit purée
- Fruit drinks and fruit juices
- Jam Grapes

5. Dairy products

- Preferably cut down on the consumption of the fattier and sugary ones.
- Full fat milk
- Fruit yogurt
- Fatty cheeses
- Milk or fruit chocolate
- Fruit-flavored yogurt drinks
- Ice cream

6. Fats

- Avoid sources of saturated fats.
- Butter
- Margarine Lard

7. Drinks

- Stay clear from those with high sugar content.
- Energy drinks
- Alcohol

- Sweetened coffee
- Carbonated soft drinks
- Sweetened tea

In addition, as a matter of thumb, you should keep to a minimum any sweets and baked goods such as croissants, cookies, etc.

This is the list of foods that you should consume in moderation to keep your prediabetes or diabetes at bay.

In the penultimate chapter, I will show you the "diabetic-friendly foods" that are your healthy allies.

6. Your "Diabetes Cookbook"

I will now tell which foods may help you prevent diabetes, regulate it, or even reverse it.

They are all foods with a low glycemic index, modest fat content, and beneficial properties for your health.

Again, I will list the foods by category.

So, here's what to prioritize in your diet to manage diabetes.

1. Carbohydrates

- Whole grains
- Brown rice
- Wholegrain pasta
- Oats

- Pasta and rice cooked al dente
- Couscous

2. Protein

- Chicken breast
- Lean cuts of red meat
- Whole eggs
- Egg whites Fish

3. Vegetables

- Vegetables are best evaluated in groups.
- Try to consume a diversity of veggies from the first groupings.
- These may be eaten raw, mildly steamed, or grilled.
- Fresh green leafy veggies (lettuce, spinach, etc.)
- Cruciferous veggies (cabbage, broccoli, etc.)
- Other Vegetables (peppers, zucchini, etc.)

Then there are root vegetables (potatoes, carrots, sweet potatoes, etc.) which are starchy therefore best minimized in your diet, and if you eat them make sure they are simply boiled or steamed.

4. Fruit

- Fresh fruit
- Oranges
- Apples
- Raspberries
- Strawberries
- Peaches
- Grapefruit
- Tangerines
- Lemons
- Frozen fruit with no added sugar

5. Dairy products

- Choose the low-fat ones.
- Skimmed milk
- Low-fat yogurt
- Light cheeses (mozzarella, ricotta, etc.)

6. Fats

Opt for excellent fat sources that are beneficial to your health.

- Extra virgin olive oil
- Foods containing omega-3s such as salmon or mackerel

7. Drinks

Choose water or unsweetened versions of Tea or Coffee for example. Or follow my recipes for healthy smoothies.

8. Bonuses

Now, let me show you 3 meals that can help you balance your blood sugar.

- **Plain live yogurt:** rich in probiotics, it helps manage blood sugar levels.
- **Chia seeds:** According to research published in the European Journal of Clinical Nutrition, they slow down the increase in sugar levels by 39%.
- **Cinnamon:** a research published in the National Library of Medicine shows how the eating of cinnamon managed to drop fasting blood sugar by between 18% and 29%.

Well, now you have learnt what foods to include in your diet to avoid, control, or revert your diabetes.

You've now reached the end of this section.

You now have a broader knowledge of diabetes, including how to manage it.

I showed you the fundamental causes of this disease — and the good practices to keep it at bay.

Next, I disclosed to you the dietary strategies to avoid diabetes or even reverse its course.

Finally, you've learned which meals to avoid — and which ones are your friends instead.

Now, you are ready to explore over 100 tasty recipes to have some delicious diabetic-friendly foods every day.

But before you do… Are you wondering how to utilize this book however, to construct a varied and balanced diet for 2000 days? Let me clarify.

I propose you eat 3 times a day with 1-2 snacks. I have offered you seafood recipes and grains and legumes recipes that may be your biggest supper each day. I have also offered you vegetable sides which may be eaten along with that main dish, so this alone offers an amazing different permutations just for your evening meal.

I have also offered you salads, soups and light dinners which are great for lunch.

Even merely going through these lunch options one by one and doing the same with the seafood, grains and legume options for your evening meal, it would be an incredible 1890 days before the same day's menu would come around again.

And then if you are picking different smoothies for breakfast too, the possibilities truly are unlimited!

GREEK YOGURT PARFAIT

- Prep Time: 5 minutes
- Cooking Time: 0 minutes
- Servings: 1

INGREDIENTS:

- 1/2 cup Greek yogurt (plain, low-fat)
- 1/4 cup fresh berries (e.g., blueberries, strawberries)
- 1 tablespoon chopped nuts (e.g., almonds, walnuts)
- 1/2 teaspoon honey (optional for sweetness)

NUTRITIONAL VALUES (APPROXIMATE):

- Calories: 200
- Carbohydrates: 20g
- Protein: 15g
- Fat: 8g
- Fiber: 3g
- Sugar: 12g

INSTRUCTIONS:

1. In a dish or glass, start with a layer of Greek yogurt.
2. Add a layer of fresh berries on top of the yogurt.
3. Sprinkle with chopped nuts for extra texture and taste.
4. If preferred, sprinkle with a tiny bit of honey for sweetness.
5. Enjoy your healthy and nutritious Greek yogurt parfait!

SCRAMBLED EGGS WITH SPINACH AND FETA

- Prep Time: 5 minutes
- Cooking Time: 10 minutes
- Servings: 2

INGREDIENTS:

- 4 big eggs
- 1 cup fresh spinach, chopped
- 1/4 cup crumbled feta cheese
- Salt and pepper to taste

NUTRITIONAL VALUES (APPROXIMATE):

- Calories: 180

- Carbohydrates: 2g

- Protein: 13g

- Fat: 14g

- Fiber: 1g

- Sugar: 1g

1. In a bowl, whisk the eggs and season with salt and pepper.

2. Heat a non-stick pan over medium heat and add spinach.

3. Cook until wilted, then pour in the eggs.

4. Scramble until thoroughly done.

5. Sprinkle with feta and serve.

OATMEAL WITH BERRIES AND ALMONDS

- Prep Time: 5 minutes

- Cooking Time: 5 minutes

- Servings: 1

INGREDIENTS:

- 1/2 cup old-fashioned oats

- 1 cup unsweetened almond milk

- 1/4 cup fresh berries

- 1 tablespoon sliced almonds

- 1/2 teaspoon cinnamon

NUTRITIONAL VALUES (APPROXIMATE):

- Calories: 250

- Carbohydrates: 35g

- Protein: 7g

- Fat: 8g

- Fiber: 7g

- Sugar: 5g

INSTRUCTIONS:

1. Combine oats and almond milk in a saucepan.

2. Heat over medium heat, stirring, until thickened.

3. Top with berries, almonds, and a sprinkling of cinnamon.

4. Please let me know if you'd want to continue with other recipes and their nutritional information.

VEGGIE OMELETTE

- Prep Time: 10 minutes
- Cooking Time: 10 minutes
- Servings: 1

INGREDIENTS:

- 2 big eggs
- 2 teaspoons diced bell peppers
- 2 tablespoons diced onions
- 2 teaspoons diced tomatoes
- Salt and pepper to taste

NUTRITIONAL VALUES (APPROXIMATE):

- Calories: 200
- Carbohydrates: 8g
- Protein: 12g
- Fat: 13g
- Fiber: 2g
- Sugar: 3g

INSTRUCTIONS:

1. In a bowl, whisk the eggs and season with salt and pepper.
2. Heat a non-stick pan over medium heat and add vegetables.
3. Pour in the whisked eggs and simmer until set.

CHIA PUDDING WITH COCONUT AND BERRIES

- Prep Time: 5 minutes (plus chilling time)
- Cooking Time: 0 minutes
- Servings: 2

INGREDIENTS:

- 1/4 cup chia seeds
- 1 cup unsweetened coconut milk
- 1/4 cup fresh berries
- 1 tablespoon shredded unsweetened coconut
- 1/2 teaspoon vanilla extract

NUTRITIONAL VALUES (APPROXIMATE):

- Calories: 180
- Carbohydrates: 13g
- Protein: 4g
- Fat: 12g
- Fiber: 8g
- Sugar: 2g

INSTRUCTIONS:

1. In a dish, blend chia seeds, coconut milk, and vanilla essence.
2. Refrigerate for a few hours or overnight until it thickens.
3. Top with fresh berries and shredded coconut before serving.

WHOLE GRAIN PANCAKES WITH SUGAR-FREE SYRUP

- Prep Time: 10 minutes
- Cooking Time: 15 minutes
- Servings: 2

INGREDIENTS:

- 1 cup whole grain pancake mix (sugar-free)
- 3/4 cup water
- Sugar-free pancake syrup (as desired)

NUTRITIONAL VALUES (APPROXIMATE):

- Calories: 200 (per serving, without syrup)
- Carbohydrates: 40g
- Protein: 7g
- Fat: 2g
- Fiber: 6g
- Sugar: 0g

INSTRUCTIONS:

1. Mix the pancake mix and water in a bowl until smooth.
2. Heat a griddle or non-stick pan over medium heat.
3. Pour the batter to create pancakes.
4. Serve with sugar-free syrup.

AVOCADO AND TOMATO TOAST ON WHOLE WHEAT BREAD

- Prep Time: 5 minutes
- Cooking Time: 0 minutes
- Servings: 1

INGREDIENTS:

- 1/2 ripe avocado, mashed 1 tiny tomato, sliced 1-piece whole wheat bread
- Salt and pepper to taste

NUTRITIONAL VALUES (APPROXIMATE):

- Calories: 220

- Carbohydrates: 23g

- Protein: 4g

- Fat: 14g

- Fiber: 7g

- Sugar: 2g

1. Toast the whole wheat bread.
2. Spread the mashed avocado on the bread.
3. Top with sliced tomatoes.
4. Season with salt and pepper.

QUINOA BREAKFAST BOWL

- Prep Time: 10 minutes
- Cooking Time: 15 minutes
- Servings: 2

INGREDIENTS:

- 1 cup cooked quinoa
- 1/2 cup unsweetened almond milk
- 1/4 cup mixed nuts and seeds (e.g., almonds, chia seeds)
- 1/2 cup fresh mixed berries
- 1/2 teaspoon honey (optional)

NUTRITIONAL VALUES (APPROXIMATE):

- Calories: 280

- Carbohydrates: 30g

- Protein: 10g

- Fat: 14g

- Fiber: 7g

- Sugar: 6g

INSTRUCTIONS:

1. In a saucepan, reheat the quinoa with almond milk.
2. Divide into bowls and top with mixed nuts, seeds, berries, and honey.

SMOKED SALMON AND CREAM CHEESE ROLL-UPS

- Prep Time: 10 minutes
- Cooking Time: 0 minutes

- Servings: 2

INGREDIENTS:

- 4 slices smoked salmon
- 4 tablespoons low-fat cream cheese
- 1 cucumber, thinly sliced
- Fresh dill for garnish

- Calories: 190
- Carbohydrates: 5g
- Protein: 12g
- Fat: 14g
- Fiber: 1g
- Sugar: 2g

1. Lay out smoked salmon slices.
2. Spread cream cheese on each piece.
3. Place cucumber slices on top.
4. Roll up and garnish with fresh dill.

COTTAGE CHEESE AND FRUIT

- Prep Time: 5 minutes
- Cooking Time: 0 minutes
- Servings: 1

- 1/2 cup low-fat cottage cheese
- 1/2 cup mixed fresh fruit (e.g., peaches, pineapple)
- 1 tablespoon chopped nuts (e.g., walnuts)

- Calories: 180
- Carbohydrates: 15g
- Protein: 15g
- Fat: 7g
- Fiber: 3g
- Sugar: 10g

1. In a bowl, put cottage cheese.
2. Top with mixed fresh fruit and chopped nuts.

SWEET POTATO HASH WITH POACHED EGGS

- Prep Time: 15 minutes
- Cooking Time: 20 minutes
- Servings: 2

- 2 medium sweet potatoes, peeled and chopped
- 1/2 onion, chopped 2 eggs
- 1 tablespoon olive oil

- Salt and pepper to taste

NUTRITIONAL VALUES (APPROXIMATE):

- Calories: 240
- Carbohydrates: 30g
- Protein: 8g
- Fat: 11g
- Fiber: 5g
- Sugar: 6g

INSTRUCTIONS:

1. Heat olive oil in a pan, add sweet potatoes and onions.
2. Sauté until sweet potatoes are soft and slightly crunchy.
3. Poach the eggs in a separate pot.
4. Serve the poached eggs on top of the sweet potato hash.

PEANUT BUTTER BANANA SMOOTHIE

- Prep Time: 5 minutes
- Cooking Time: 0 minutes
- Servings: 1

INGREDIENTS:

- 1 ripe banana
- 2 teaspoons natural peanut butter
- 1 cup unsweetened almond milk
- 1/2 teaspoon cinnamon
- Ice cubes (optional)

NUTRITIONAL VALUES (APPROXIMATE):

- Calories: 320
- Carbohydrates: 31g
- Protein: 9g
- Fat: 20g
- Fiber: 6g
- Sugar: 14g

INSTRUCTIONS:

1. Place banana, peanut butter, almond milk, and cinnamon in a blender.
2. Blend until smooth. Add ice cubes if desired.

SPINACH AND MUSHROOM QUICHE

- Prep Time: 15 minutes
- Cooking Time: 40 minutes
- Servings: 6

INGREDIENTS:

- 1 premade whole wheat pie crust
- 4 big eggs

- 1 cup fresh spinach, chopped
- 1 cup sliced mushrooms
- 1/2 cup low-fat milk
- Salt and pepper to taste

NUTRITIONAL VALUES (APPROXIMATE):

- Calories: 220 (per serving)
- Carbohydrates: 18g
- Protein: 9g
- Fat: 13g
- Fiber: 3g

- Sugar: 3g

INSTRUCTIONS:

1. Preheat oven to 375°F (190°C).
2. In a pan, sauté mushrooms and spinach until softened.
3. In a bowl, mix eggs, milk, salt, and pepper.
4. Place the sautéed veggies in the pie shell, pour egg mixture over them.
5. Bake for approximately 40 minutes or until set.

OVERNIGHT OATS WITH APPLE AND CINNAMON

- Prep Time: 5 minutes (plus chilling time)
- Cooking Time: 0 minutes
- Servings: 1

INGREDIENTS:

- 1/2 cup old-fashioned oats
- 1/2 cup unsweetened almond milk
- 1 small apple, diced
- 1/2 teaspoon cinnamon
- 1 tablespoon chopped nuts (e.g., almonds, pecans)

NUTRITIONAL VALUES (APPROXIMATE):

- Calories: 280
- Carbohydrates: 46g
- Protein: 6g
- Fat: 8g
- Fiber: 9g
- Sugar: 17g

INSTRUCTIONS:

1. In a container, mix oats, almond milk, chopped apple, and cinnamon.
2. Refrigerate overnight.
3. Top with chopped nuts before serving

TOFU SCRAMBLE WITH VEGGIES

- Prep Time: 10 minutes
- Cooking Time: 15 minutes
- Servings: 2

INGREDIENTS:

- 1/2 brick of firm tofu, crumbled
- 1/2 cup chopped bell peppers
- 1/2 cup diced onions
- 1/2 cup chopped tomatoes
- 1/2 teaspoon turmeric
- Salt and pepper to taste

NUTRITIONAL VALUES (APPROXIMATE):

- Calories: 160 (per serving)
- Carbohydrates: 10g
- Protein: 12g
- Fat: 8g
- Fiber: 3g
- Sugar: 4g

INSTRUCTIONS:

1. In a pan, sauté onions, bell peppers, and tomatoes.
2. Add crumbled tofu and turmeric.
3. Cook until heated through and season with salt and pepper.

ALMOND FLOUR WAFFLES

- Prep Time: 10 minutes
- Cooking Time: 10 minutes
- Servings: 2

INGREDIENTS:

- 1 cup almond flour
- 2 eggs
- 1/4 cup unsweetened almond milk
- 1/2 teaspoon baking powder
- 1/2 teaspoon vanilla extract

NUTRITIONAL VALUES (APPROXIMATE):

- Calories: 220 (per serving)
- Carbohydrates: 6g
- Protein: 9g
- Fat: 18g
- Fiber: 3g
- Sugar: 1g

INSTRUCTIONS:

1. In a dish, combine almond flour, eggs, almond milk, baking powder, and vanilla extract.

2. Preheat waffle iron and pour batter to create waffles.

BAKED AVOCADO EGGS

- Prep Time: 5 minutes
- Cooking Time: 15 minutes
- Servings: 2

INGREDIENTS:

- 2 ripe avocados
- 4 eggs
- Salt and pepper to taste
- Chopped fresh herbs for garnish (e.g., parsley, chives)

NUTRITIONAL VALUES (APPROXIMATE):

- Calories: 220 (per serving)
- Carbohydrates: 9g
- Protein: 7g
- Fat: 18g
- Fiber: 7g
- Sugar: 1g

INSTRUCTIONS:

1. Preheat oven to 375°F (190°C).
2. Cut avocados in half and scrape out a little flesh.
3. Crack one egg into each avocado half.
4. Season with salt and pepper.
5. Bake for approximately 15 minutes or until the eggs are set.

GARNISH WITH CHOPPED HERBS.

- Prep Time: 5 minutes
- Cooking Time: 0 minutes
- Servings: 1

INGREDIENTS:

- 2 slices whole grain bread
- 2 tablespoons low-fat cream cheese
- 4-5 cucumber slices
- Fresh dill for garnish

NUTRITIONAL VALUES (APPROXIMATE):

- Calories: 190

- Carbohydrates: 25g

- Protein: 6g

- Fat: 7g

- Fiber: 4g

- Sugar: 3g

INSTRUCTIONS:

1. Spread cream cheese on one piece of bread.

2. Layer cucumber slices on top.

3. Garnish with fresh dill.

4. Top with the second piece of bread.

VEGGIE BREAKFAST BURRITO

- Prep Time: 15 minutes
- Cooking Time: 10 minutes
- Servings: 2

INGREDIENTS:

- 4 whole grain tortillas

- 4 big eggs

- 1/2 cup chopped bell peppers

- 1/2 cup diced onions

- Salsa (optional)

- Salt and pepper to taste

NUTRITIONAL VALUES (APPROXIMATE):

- Calories: 300 (per burrito)

- Carbohydrates: 40g

- Protein: 15g

- Fat: 10g

- Fiber: 8g

- Sugar: 4g

INSTRUCTIONS:

1. Scramble the eggs and season with salt and pepper.

2. In a pan, sauté onions and bell peppers.

3. Warm tortillas and fill with scrambled eggs and sautéed vegetables.

4. Add salsa if desired and roll into a tortilla.

BROCCOLI AND CHEDDAR EGG MUFFINS

- ✦ **Prep Time: 10 minutes**
- ✦ **Cooking Time: 25 minutes**
- ✦ **Servings: 6 muffins**

INGREDIENTS:

- 6 big eggs
- 1 cup chopped broccoli
- 1/2 cup shredded low-fat cheddar cheese
- Salt and pepper to taste

NUTRITIONAL VALUES (APPROXIMATE):

- Calories: 130 (per muffin)
- Carbohydrates: 3g
- Protein: 10g
- Fat: 9g
- Fiber: 1g
- Sugar: 1g

INSTRUCTIONS:

1. Preheat the oven to 350°F (175°C) and oil a muffin tray.
2. In a bowl, whisk the eggs and season with salt and pepper.
3. Stir in chopped broccoli and cheddar cheese.
4. Pour the mixture into the muffin tray.
5. Bake for approximately 25 minutes or until the muffins are set.

SESAME SEEDS FISH FILLET

- Prep Time: 10 minutes
- Cooking Time: 15 minutes
- Servings: 2

INGREDIENTS:

- 2 fish fillets (e.g., tilapia, cod)
- 2 teaspoons sesame seeds
- 2 tablespoons olive oil
- 1 lemon, juiced
- Salt and pepper to taste

NUTRITIONAL VALUES (APPROXIMATE):

- Calories: 250 (per serving)
- Carbohydrates: 3g
- Protein: 25g
- Fat: 16g
- Fiber: 2g
- Sugar: 1g

INSTRUCTIONS:

1. Preheat the oven to 375°F (190°C).
2. Season fish fillets with salt and pepper, then cover with sesame seeds.
3. Heat olive oil in an ovenproof skillet.
4. Sear fish fillets on both sides for 2-3 minutes.
5. Transfer the skillet to the oven and bake for approximately 10 minutes.
6. Drizzle with lemon juice before serving.

BACON-WRAPPED SHRIMPS

- Prep Time: 15 minutes
- Cooking Time: 10 minutes
- Servings: 4

INGREDIENTS:

- 16 big shrimp, peeled and deveined
- 8 pieces of bacon
- 1/4 cup maple syrup
- Wooden toothpicks

NUTRITIONAL VALUES (APPROXIMATE):

- Calories: 160 (per serving, 4 shrimps)
- Carbohydrates: 8g
- Protein: 10g
- Fat: 10g

- Fiber: 0g
- Sugar: 5g

INSTRUCTIONS:

1. Preheat the oven to 400°F (200°C).

2. Wrap each shrimp with a piece of bacon and fasten with toothpicks.
3. Place the bacon-wrapped shrimps on a baking sheet.
4. Brush with maple syrup.
5. Bake for approximately 10 minutes or until the bacon is crispy.

LEMON PEPPER SHRIMP IN AIR FRYER

- Prep Time: 10 minutes
- Cooking Time: 10 minutes
- Servings: 2

INGREDIENTS:

- 1/2-pound big shrimp, peeled and deveined
- 2 tablespoons olive oil
- 1 lemon, juiced and zested
- 1 teaspoon black pepper
- Salt to taste

NUTRITIONAL VALUES (APPROXIMATE):

- Calories: 180 (per serving)
- Carbohydrates: 3g
- Protein: 22g
- Fat: 9g
- Fiber: 1g
- Sugar: 1g

INSTRUCTIONS:

1. In a bowl, combine olive oil, lemon juice, lemon zest, black pepper, and a bit of salt.
2. Toss shrimp in the mixture and let them marinade for a few minutes.
3. Place shrimp in the air fryer basket and cook at 375°F (190°C) for approximately 10 minutes or until they become pink.

MONK-FISH CURRY

- Prep Time: 15 minutes
- Cooking Time: 20 minutes
- Servings: 4

INGREDIENTS:

- 1-pound monkfish fillets, cut into portions
- 1 onion, chopped 2 cloves garlic, minced
- 2 tablespoons curry paste (of your choice)
- 1 can (14 Oz) coconut milk
- 1 red bell pepper, sliced 2 tablespoons vegetable oil
- Salt and pepper to taste

NUTRITIONAL VALUES (APPROXIMATE):

- Calories: 300 (per serving)
- Carbohydrates: 8g
- Protein: 25g
- Fat: 20g
- Fiber: 3g
- Sugar: 4g

INSTRUCTIONS:

1. Heat vegetable oil in a large pan and sauté onions and garlic.
2. Add curry paste and cook for a minute.
3. Stir in coconut milk and bring to a boil.
4. Add monkfish and bell peppers, then boil until fish is cooked through.
5. Season with salt and pepper.

LEMON SALMON WITH KAFFIR LIME

- 2 tablespoons olive oil
- Salt and pepper to taste

- Prep Time: 10 minutes
- Cooking Time: 15 minutes
- Servings: 2

INGREDIENTS:

- 2 salmon fillets
- 2 kaffir lime leaves, coarsely chopped
- 1 lemon, juiced and zested

NUTRITIONAL VALUES (APPROXIMATE):

- Calories: 250 (per serving)
- Carbohydrates: 2g
- Protein: 25g

- Fat: 16g
- Fiber: 1g
- Sugar: 1g

INSTRUCTIONS:

1. Preheat the oven to 375°F (190°C).

2. In a bowl, combine olive oil, lemon juice, lemon zest, kaffir lime leaves, salt, and pepper.

3. Place salmon fillets in a baking dish and pour the mixture over them.

4. Bake for approximately 15 minutes or until the fish flakes easily.

BAKED FISH SERVED WITH VEGETABLES

- **Prep Time: 15 minutes**
- **Cooking Time: 25 minutes**
- **Servings: 4**

INGREDIENTS:

- 4 fish fillets (e.g., cod, haddock)
- 2 zucchinis, sliced 2 tomatoes, sliced 1 lemon, sliced 2 cloves garlic, minced 2 tablespoons olive oil
- Salt and pepper to taste

NUTRITIONAL VALUES (APPROXIMATE):

- Calories: 220 (per serving)
- Carbohydrates: 10g
- Protein: 25g
- Fat: 8g
- Fiber: 3g
- Sugar: 5g

INSTRUCTIONS:

1. Preheat the oven to 375°F (190°C).

2. Place fish fillets on a baking sheet and season with salt, pepper, and chopped garlic.

3. Arrange sliced zucchinis, tomatoes, and lemon on top.

4. Drizzle with olive oil.

5. Bake for approximately 25 minutes or until the fish is done and the vegetables are soft.

+ **Prep Time: 15 minutes**
+ **Cooking Time: 25 minutes**
+ **Servings: 4**

INGREDIENTS:

- 4 fish fillets (e.g., snapper, grouper)
- 2 cups mixed veggies (e.g., broccoli, carrots, bell peppers)
- 2 tablespoons olive oil
- 2 cloves garlic, minced
- 1 teaspoon dry herbs (e.g., thyme, rosemary)
- Salt and pepper to taste

NUTRITIONAL VALUES (APPROXIMATE):

- Calories: 280 (per serving)
- Carbohydrates: 12g
- Protein: 28g
- Fat: 14g
- Fiber: 4g
- Sugar: 4g

INSTRUCTIONS:

1. Preheat the oven to 375°F (190°C).
2. Toss mixed veggies with olive oil, garlic, dried herbs, salt, and pepper.
3. Spread veggies on a baking sheet.
4. Place fish fillets on top of the veggies.
5. Bake for approximately 25 minutes or until the fish flakes easily.

SPICY COD

+ **Prep Time: 10 minutes**
+ **Cooking Time: 15 minutes**
+ **Servings: 2**

INGREDIENTS:

- 2 cod fillets
- 2 tablespoons chili powder
- 1 teaspoon paprika
- 1/2 teaspoon cumin
- 1/4 teaspoon cayenne pepper
- 2 tablespoons olive oil
- Salt and pepper to taste

NUTRITIONAL VALUES (APPROXIMATE):

- Calories: 230 (per serving)
- Carbohydrates: 3g
- Protein: 30g
- Fat: 11g
- Fiber: 1g
- Sugar: 1g

INSTRUCTIONS:

1. Preheat the oven to 375°F (190°C).
2. In a small bowl, add chili powder, paprika, cumin, cayenne pepper, salt, and pepper.
3. Rub the spice mixture on both sides of fish fillets.
4. Heat olive oil in an ovenproof skillet.
5. Sear cod fillets for a minute on each side.
6. Transfer the skillet to the oven and bake for around 12-15 minutes.

STEAMED BLUE CRABS

- Prep Time: 15 minutes
- Cooking Time: 25 minutes
- Servings: 4

INGREDIENTS:

- 8 live blue crabs
- 1 cup water
- 1 cup white vinegar
- 2 bay leaves
- 2 teaspoons Old Bay seasoning
- Butter for dipping

NUTRITIONAL VALUES (APPROXIMATE):

- Calories: 120 (per crab, without butter)
- Carbohydrates: 1g Protein: 22g
- Fat: 2g
- Fiber: 0g
- Sugar: 0g

INSTRUCTIONS:

1. In a big saucepan, bring water, vinegar, bay leaves, and Old Bay seasoning to a boil.
2. Place a steamer basket in the pot.
3. Add live blue crabs and cover.
4. Steam for approximately 20-25 minutes or until they become bright orange.
5. Serve with melted butter for dipping.

- ↓ **Prep Time: 15 minutes**
- ↓ **Cooking Time: 15 minutes**
- ↓ **Servings: 2**

INGREDIENTS:

- 2 salmon fillets
- 2 tablespoons soy sauce (low-sodium)
- 1 tablespoon sesame oil
- 1 tablespoon fresh ginger, grated
- 1 clove garlic, minced
- 1 tablespoon sesame seeds
- Salt and pepper to taste

NUTRITIONAL VALUES (APPROXIMATE):

- Calories: 300 (per serving)
- Carbohydrates: 3g
- Protein: 25g
- Fat: 20g
- Fiber: 1g
- Sugar: 0g

INSTRUCTIONS:

1. In a bowl, combine soy sauce, sesame oil, ginger, garlic, and a touch of salt and pepper.
2. Marinate the salmon in the marinade for a few minutes.
3. Preheat a pan or grill and cook the salmon fillets for approximately 6-7 minutes on each side, basting with the marinade.
4. Sprinkle sesame seeds before serving.

- ↓ **Prep Time: 15 minutes**
- ↓ **Cooking Time: 15 minutes**
- ↓ **Servings: 4**

INGREDIENTS:

- 8 ounces' whole wheat spaghetti
- 2 cans (5 Oz each) tuna in water, drained
- 2 tablespoons olive oil
- 2 cloves garlic, minced 1/2 cup cherry tomatoes, halved
- 1/4 cup fresh basil leaves
- Salt and pepper to taste

NUTRITIONAL VALUES (APPROXIMATE):

- Calories: 250 (per serving)
- Carbohydrates: 30g

- Protein: 20g
- Fat: 7g
- Fiber: 5g
- Sugar: 2g

INSTRUCTIONS:

1. Cook the pasta according per package directions.
2. In a pan, heat olive oil and sauté garlic.
3. Add tuna and cherry tomatoes, simmering for a few minutes.
4. Toss the cooked spaghetti and fresh basil into the skillet.
5. Season with salt and pepper before serving.

TUNA SWEETCORN CASSEROLE

- Prep Time: 15 minutes
- Cooking Time: 30 minutes
- Servings: 4

INGREDIENTS:

- 2 cans (5 Oz each) tuna in water, drained
- 1 cup frozen sweetcorn
- 1/2 cup low-fat mayonnaise
- 1/2 cup low-fat cheddar cheese, shredded
- 2 teaspoons whole wheat breadcrumbs

NUTRITIONAL VALUES (APPROXIMATE):

- Calories: 220 (per serving)
- Carbohydrates: 10g
- Protein: 20g
- Fat: 11g
- Fiber: 2g
- Sugar: 2g

INSTRUCTIONS:

1. Preheat the oven to 375°F (190°C).
2. In a bowl, mix tuna, sweetcorn, and mayonnaise.
3. Transfer to a baking dish and sprinkle with shredded cheddar and breadcrumbs.
4. Bake for approximately 30 minutes or until the top is brown and bubbling.

SWORDFISH STEAK

- Prep Time: 10 minutes
- Cooking Time: 10 minutes
- Servings: 2

INGREDIENTS:

- 2 swordfish steaks
- 2 tablespoons olive oil
- 1 lemon, juiced and zested
- 2 cloves garlic, minced
- 1 teaspoon dried oregano
- Salt and pepper to taste

NUTRITIONAL VALUES (APPROXIMATE):

- Calories: 280 (per serving)
- Carbohydrates: 3g
- Protein: 30g
- Fat: 16g
- Fiber: 1g
- Sugar: 1g

INSTRUCTIONS:

1. Preheat the grill or a grill pan.
2. In a bowl, combine olive oil, lemon juice, lemon zest, garlic, oregano, salt, and pepper.
3. Brush the swordfish steaks with the mixture.
4. Grill for approximately 4-5 minutes on each side or until cooked through.

TARRAGON COD FILLETS

- **Prep Time: 15 minutes**
- **Cooking Time: 15 minutes**
- **Servings: 2**

INGREDIENTS:

- 2 cod fillets
- 1/4 cup plain Greek yogurt
- 1 tablespoon fresh tarragon, chopped 1 lemon, juiced
- Salt and pepper to taste

NUTRITIONAL VALUES (APPROXIMATE):

- Calories: 190 (per serving)
- Carbohydrates: 5g
- Protein: 30g
- Fat: 4g
- Fiber: 0g
- Sugar: 2g

INSTRUCTIONS:

1. Preheat the oven to 375°F (190°C).
2. In a bowl, combine Greek yogurt, tarragon, lemon juice, salt, and pepper.
3. Place fish fillets in a baking dish and sprinkle the yogurt mixture on top.
4. Bake for approximately 15 minutes or until the fish flakes easily.

SESAME SHRIMP MIX

- ⚜ **Prep Time: 10 minutes**
- ⚜ **Cooking Time: 10 minutes**
- ⚜ **Servings: 2**

INGREDIENTS:

- 1/2-pound big shrimp, peeled and deveined
- 2 tablespoons soy sauce (low-sodium)
- 1 tablespoon sesame oil
- 1 tablespoon sesame seeds
- 1 tablespoon green onions, chopped
- Salt and pepper to taste

NUTRITIONAL VALUES (APPROXIMATE):

- Calories: 180 (per serving)
- Carbohydrates: 3g
- Protein: 22g
- Fat: 9g
- Fiber: 1g
- Sugar: 0g

INSTRUCTIONS:

1. In a bowl, combine soy sauce, sesame oil, sesame seeds, green onions, salt, and pepper.
2. Toss shrimp in the mixture and let them marinade for a few minutes.
3. Heat a skillet and cook the shrimp for approximately 2-3 minutes on each side.

CAULIFLOWER MASHED POTATOES

- Prep Time: 15 minutes
- Cooking Time: 15 minutes
- Servings: 4

INGREDIENTS:

- 1 medium head of cauliflower, chopped into florets
- 2 cloves garlic, minced
- 2 tablespoons low-fat sour cream
- Salt and pepper to taste

NUTRITIONAL VALUES (APPROXIMATE):

- Calories: 80 (per serving)
- Carbohydrates: 15g
- Protein: 6g
- Fat: 1g
- Fiber: 6g
- Sugar: 5g

INSTRUCTIONS:

1. Steam or boil cauliflower florets until soft.
2. In a food processor, combine
3. cauliflower with minced garlic, sour cream, salt, and pepper until smoot

ROASTED TOMATO BRUSSELS SPROUTS

- Prep Time: 10 minutes
- Cooking Time: 25 minutes
- Servings: 4

INGREDIENTS:

- 1 pound Brussels sprouts, trimmed and halved

- 1 cup cherry tomatoes
- 2 tablespoons olive oil
- Salt and pepper to taste

NUTRITIONAL VALUES (APPROXIMATE):

- Calories: 100 (per serving)

- Carbohydrates: 10g

- Protein: 3g

- Fat: 6g

- Fiber: 4g

- Sugar: 3g

INSTRUCTIONS:

1. Preheat the oven to 400°F (200°C).

2. Toss Brussels sprouts and cherry tomatoes with olive oil, salt, and pepper.

3. Roast for approximately 20-25 minutes or until tender and slightly browned.

SIMPLE SAUTÉED GREENS

- Prep Time: 10 minutes
- Cooking Time: 10 minutes
- Servings: 4

INGREDIENTS:

- 1 bunch of your favorite greens (e.g., spinach, kale, chard)

- 2 cloves garlic, minced

- 2 tablespoons olive oil

- Lemon juice to taste

- Salt and pepper to taste

NUTRITIONAL VALUES (APPROXIMATE):

- Calories: 40 (per serving)

- Carbohydrates: 3g

- Protein: 2g

- Fat: 3g

- Fiber: 2g

- Sugar: 1g

INSTRUCTIONS:

1. Heat olive oil in a large pan and sauté minced garlic.

2. Add greens and simmer until wilted.

3. Season with lemon juice, salt, and pepper.

GREEN BEANS IN OVEN

- ↓ **Prep Time: 10 minutes**
- ↓ **Cooking Time: 20 minutes**
- ↓ **Servings: 4**

INGREDIENTS:

- 1 pound fresh green beans, trimmed
- 2 tablespoons olive oil
- 2 cloves garlic, minced
- Salt and pepper to taste

NUTRITIONAL VALUES (APPROXIMATE):

- Calories: 70 (per serving)
- Carbohydrates: 6g
- Protein: 2g
- Fat: 5g
- Fiber: 2g
- Sugar: 2g

INSTRUCTIONS:

1. Preheat the oven to 400°F (200°C).
2. Toss green beans with olive oil, minced garlic, salt, and pepper.
3. Roast for approximately 15-20 minutes or until tender and slightly crunchy.

GREEN BEANS WITH PAPRIKA

VALUES (APPROXIMATE):

- ↓ **Prep Time: 10 minutes**
- ↓ **Cooking Time: 15 minutes**
- ↓ **Servings: 4**

INGREDIENTS:

- 1 pound fresh green beans, trimmed
- 1 teaspoon paprika
- 2 tablespoons olive oil
- Salt and pepper to taste

- Calories: 80 (per serving)
- Carbohydrates: 6g
- Protein: 2g
- Fat: 6g
- Fiber: 3g
- Sugar: 2g

INSTRUCTIONS:

1. Heat olive oil in a skillet.
2. Add green beans and paprika, sauté until cooked.
3. Season with salt and pepper.

ROSEMARY POTATOES

- Prep Time: 15 minutes
- Cooking Time: 25 minutes
- Servings: 4

INGREDIENTS:

- 1-pound baby potatoes
- 2 tablespoons olive oil
- 1 tablespoon fresh rosemary, chopped
- Salt and pepper to taste

NUTRITIONAL VALUES (APPROXIMATE):

- Calories: 120 (per serving)
- Carbohydrates: 15g
- Protein: 2g
- Fat: 6g
- Fiber: 2g
- Sugar: 1g

INSTRUCTIONS:

1. Preheat the oven to 400°F (200°C).
2. Toss baby potatoes with olive oil, fresh rosemary, salt, and pepper.
3. Roast for approximately 20-25 minutes or until potatoes are soft and golden.

CORN ON THE COB

- Prep Time: 5 minutes
- Cooking Time: 10 minutes
- Servings: 4

INGREDIENTS:

- 4 ears of fresh corn
- Butter or olive oil (as desired)
- Salt and pepper to taste

NUTRITIONAL VALUES (APPROXIMATE):

- Calories: 80 (per serving)
- Carbohydrates: 18g
- Protein: 2g
- Fat: 1g
- Fiber: 2g
- Sugar: 4g

INSTRUCTIONS:

1. Boil or grill the corn until soft.
2. Serve with butter or olive oil and season with salt and pepper.

MASHED PUMPKIN

- Prep Time: 15 minutes
- Cooking Time: 20 minutes
- Servings: 4

INGREDIENTS:

- 1 small pumpkin, peeled and cubed
- 2 tablespoons low-fat sour cream
- 1 tablespoon fresh thyme leaves
- Salt and pepper to taste

NUTRITIONAL VALUES (APPROXIMATE):

- Calories: 90 (per serving)
- Carbohydrates: 20g
- Protein: 2g
- Fat: 1g
- Fiber: 4g
- Sugar: 5g

INSTRUCTIONS:

1. Steam or boil pumpkin chunks until soft.
2. Mash the pumpkin and blend with low-fat sour cream, fresh thyme, salt, and pepper.

AROMATIC TOASTED PUMPKIN SEEDS

- Prep Time: 5 minutes
- Cooking Time: 10 minutes
- Servings: 4

INGREDIENTS:

- 1 cup pumpkin seeds (cleaned and dried)
- 1/2 teaspoon olive oil
- 1/2 teaspoon ground cumin
- 1/2 teaspoon paprika
- Salt to taste

NUTRITIONAL VALUES (APPROXIMATE):

- Calories: 90 (per serving)
- Carbohydrates: 2g
- Protein: 4g
- Fat: 7g
- Fiber: 1g

- Sugar: 0g

INSTRUCTIONS:

1. Preheat the oven to 350°F (175°C).

2. Toss pumpkin seeds with olive oil, ground cumin, paprika, and a touch of salt.

3. Spread the seeds on a baking sheet and roast for approximately 10 minutes or until they become brown.

BALSAMIC CABBAGE

- Prep Time: 10 minutes
- Cooking Time: 15 minutes
- Servings: 4

INGREDIENTS:

- 1 small head of cabbage, thinly sliced
- 2 tablespoons balsamic vinegar
- 1 tablespoon olive oil
- 1 teaspoon honey
- Salt and pepper to taste

NUTRITIONAL VALUES (APPROXIMATE):

- Calories: 60 (per serving)
- Carbohydrates: 9g
- Protein: 1g
- Fat: 3g
- Fiber: 4g
- Sugar: 5g

INSTRUCTIONS:

1. In a large skillet, heat olive oil.
2. Add cabbage and sauté until it starts to soften.
3. Stir in balsamic vinegar, honey, salt, and pepper.
4. Continue cooking for a few more minutes until the cabbage is soft.

CHILI BROCCOLI

- Prep Time: 10 minutes
- Cooking Time: 15 minutes
- Servings: 4

INGREDIENTS:

- 1-pound broccoli florets
- 2 tablespoons olive oil

- 1/2 teaspoon chili powder
- Salt and pepper to taste

NUTRITIONAL VALUES (APPROXIMATE):

- Calories: 70 (per serving)
- Carbohydrates: 6g
- Protein: 2g
- Fat: 5g
- Fiber: 3g

- Sugar: 2g

INSTRUCTIONS:

1. Preheat the oven to 400°F (200°C).
2. Toss broccoli florets with olive oil, chili powder, salt, and pepper.
3. Roast for approximately 15 minutes or until the broccoli is soft and slightly crunchy.

PAPRIKA BRUSSELS SPROUTS

- Prep Time: 10 minutes
- Cooking Time: 20 minutes
- Servings: 4

INGREDIENTS:

- 1 pound Brussels sprouts, trimmed and halved
- 2 tablespoons olive oil
- 1 teaspoon paprika
- Salt and pepper to taste

NUTRITIONAL VALUES (APPROXIMATE):

- Calories: 80 (per serving)
- Carbohydrates: 8g
- Protein: 3g
- Fat: 5g
- Fiber: 4g
- Sugar: 2g

INSTRUCTIONS:

1. Preheat the oven to 400°F (200°C).
2. Toss Brussels sprouts with olive oil, paprika, salt, and pepper.
3. Roast for approximately 15-20 minutes or until tender and slightly browned.

SPICY BRUSSELS SPROUTS

- Prep Time: 10 minutes
- Cooking Time: 20 minutes

- Servings: 4

INGREDIENTS:

- 1 pound Brussels sprouts, trimmed and halved
- 2 tablespoons olive oil
- 1/2 teaspoon red pepper flakes
- Salt and pepper to taste

NUTRITIONAL VALUES (APPROXIMATE):

- Calories: 70 (per serving)
- Carbohydrates: 7g
- Protein: 3g
- Fat: 5g
- Fiber: 3g
- Sugar: 2g

INSTRUCTIONS:

1. Preheat the oven to 400°F (200°C).
2. Toss Brussels sprouts with olive oil, red pepper flakes, salt, and pepper.
3. Roast for approximately 15-20 minutes or until tender and slightly crunchy.

BAKED CAULIFLOWER WITH CHILI

- Prep Time: 10 minutes
- Cooking Time: 20 minutes
- Servings: 4

INGREDIENTS:

- 1 head of cauliflower, chopped into florets
- 2 tablespoons olive oil
- 1 teaspoon chili powder
- Salt and pepper to taste

NUTRITIONAL VALUES (APPROXIMATE):

- Calories: 60 (per serving)
- Carbohydrates: 7g
- Protein: 3g
- Fat: 5g
- Fiber: 3g
- Sugar: 3g

INSTRUCTIONS:

1. Preheat the oven to 400°F (200°C).
2. Toss cauliflower florets with olive oil, chili powder, salt, and pepper.
3. Roast for approximately 15-20 minutes or until the cauliflower is soft and slightly browned.

ROASTED BRUSSELS SPROUTS

- Prep Time: 10 minutes
- Cooking Time: 20 minutes
- Servings: 4

INGREDIENTS:

- 1 pound Brussels sprouts, trimmed and halved
- 2 tablespoons balsamic vinegar
- 1 tablespoon olive oil
- Salt and pepper to taste

NUTRITIONAL VALUES (APPROXIMATE):

- Calories: 70 (per serving)
- Carbohydrates: 9g
- Protein: 3g
- Fat: 3g
- Fiber: 4g
- Sugar: 2g

INSTRUCTIONS:

1. Preheat the oven to 400°F (200°C).
2. Toss Brussels sprouts with balsamic vinegar, olive oil, salt, and pepper.
3. Roast for approximately 15-20 minutes or until tender and slightly browned.

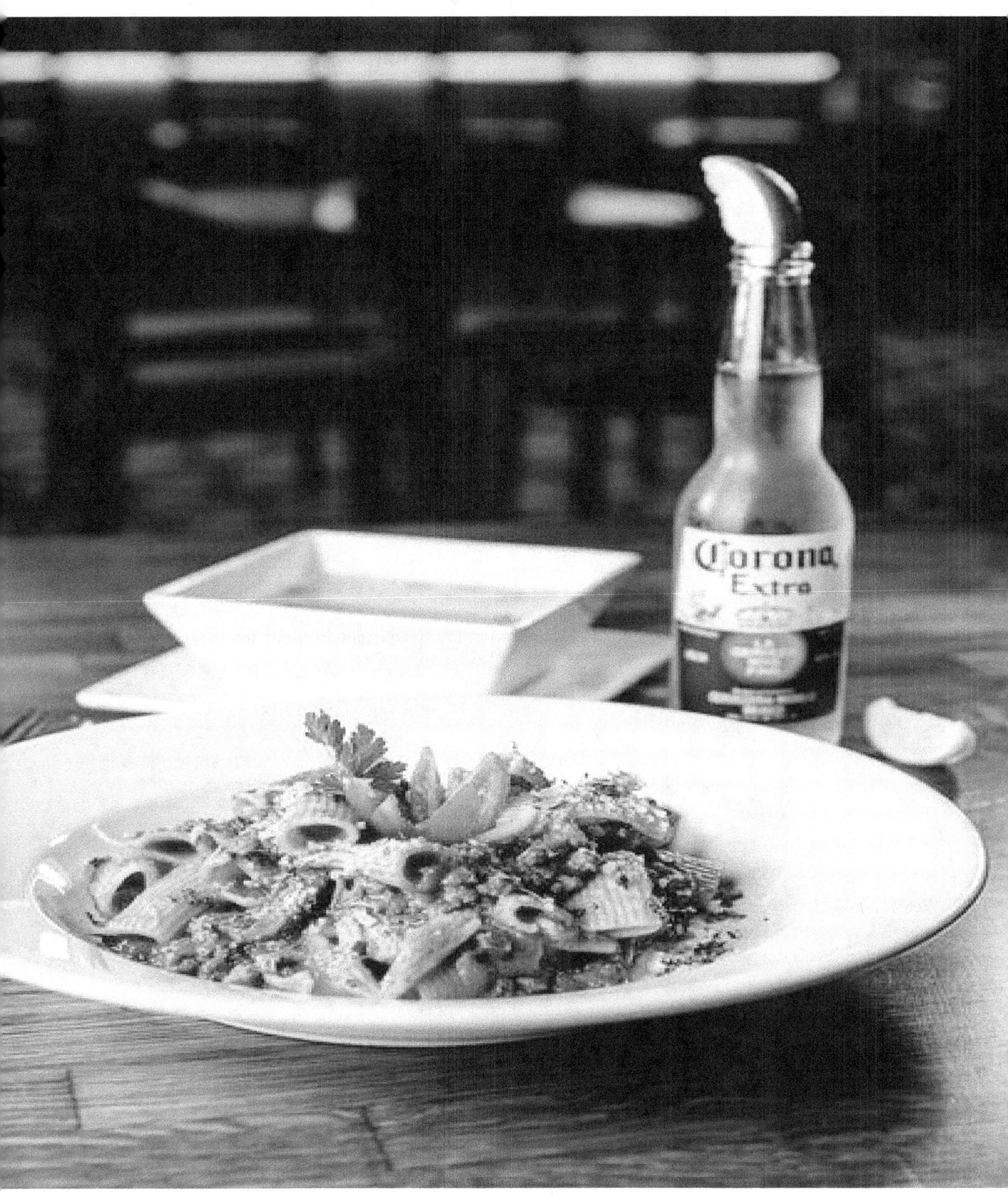

SEASONED WILD RICE

- Prep Time: 10 minutes
- Cooking Time: 45 minutes
- Servings: 4

INGREDIENTS:

- 1 cup wild rice
- 2 cups water or vegetable broth
- 1/2 teaspoon dried thyme
- 1/2 teaspoon dried rosemary
- Salt and pepper to taste

NUTRITIONAL VALUES (APPROXIMATE):

- Calories: 150 (per serving)
- Carbohydrates: 30g
- Protein: 4g
- Fat: 0.5g
- Fiber: 3g
- Sugar: 0g

INSTRUCTIONS:

1. In a saucepan, add wild rice, water or vegetable broth, thyme, rosemary, salt, and pepper.
2. Bring to a boil, then decrease the heat, cover, and simmer for approximately 45 minutes or until the rice is soft and the liquid is absorbed.

QUINOA

- Prep Time: 5 minutes
- Cooking Time: 15 minutes
- Servings: 4

INGREDIENTS:

- 1 cup quinoa
- 2 cups water or vegetable broth
- Salt to taste

NUTRITIONAL VALUES (APPROXIMATE):

- Calories: 180 (per serving)
- Carbohydrates: 30g
- Protein: 6g
- Fat: 3.5g
- Fiber: 3g
- Sugar: 0g

INSTRUCTIONS:

1. Rinse quinoa in cool water.

2. In a saucepan, add quinoa, water or vegetable broth, and a bit of salt.

3. Bring to a boil, then decrease the heat, cover, and simmer for approximately 15 minutes or until the quinoa is cooked and the liquid is absorbed.

MILLET TABBOULEH, LIME, AND CILANTRO

- Prep Time: 15 minutes
- Cooking Time: 20 minutes
- Servings: 4

INGREDIENTS:

- 1 cup millet
- 2 cups water or vegetable broth
- 1/4 cup fresh cilantro, chopped Juice of 2 limes
- Salt and pepper to taste

NUTRITIONAL VALUES (APPROXIMATE):

- Calories: 160 (per serving)
- Carbohydrates: 35g
- Protein: 5g
- Fat: 1g
- Fiber: 4g
- Sugar: 0g

INSTRUCTIONS:

1. In a saucepan, mix millet, water or vegetable broth, and a bit of salt.

2. Bring to a boil, then decrease the heat, cover, and simmer for approximately 20 minutes or until the millet is cooked and the liquid is absorbed.

3. Fluff the millet with a fork and toss in cilantro, lime juice, salt, and pepper.

GRILLED TOFU WITH SESAME SEEDS

- Prep Time: 10 minutes
- Cooking Time: 10 minutes
- Servings: 4

INGREDIENTS:

- 1 brick of firm tofu, cut
- 2 tablespoons soy sauce (low-sodium)
- 1 tablespoon sesame oil
- 1 tablespoon sesame seeds
- Salt and pepper to taste

NUTRITIONAL VALUES (APPROXIMATE):

- Calories: 180 (per serving)
- Carbohydrates: 4g
- Protein: 12g
- Fat: 12g
- Fiber: 2g
- Sugar: 1g

INSTRUCTIONS:

1. Preheat a grill or grill pan.
2. Marinate tofu slices in a combination of soy sauce, sesame oil, salt, and pepper for a few minutes.
3. Grill tofu slices for approximately 5 side, putting sesame seeds on top.

OUTHWEST TOFU SCRAMBLE

- Prep Time: 10 minutes
- Cooking Time: 15 minutes
- Servings: 4

INGREDIENTS:

- 1 brick of firm tofu, crumbled
- 1/2 red bell pepper, diced 1/2 red onion, diced
- 1 teaspoon chili powder
- 1/2 teaspoon cumin
- Salt and pepper to taste

NUTRITIONAL VALUES (APPROXIMATE):

- Calories: 160 (per serving)
- Carbohydrates: 10g
- Protein: 13g
- Fat: 7g
- Fiber: 3g
- Sugar: 3g

INSTRUCTIONS:

1. In a pan, sauté red bell pepper and red onion until softened.
2. Add crumbled tofu, chili powder, cumin, salt, and pepper.
3. Cook until tofu is cooked through and seasonings are fully integrated.

BLACK-BEAN AND VEGETABLE BURRITO

- Prep Time: 15 minutes
- Cooking Time: 15 minutes
- Servings: 4

INGREDIENTS:

- 1 can (15 Oz) black beans, drained and rinsed

- 1 cup mixed veggies (e.g., bell peppers, maize, onions)
- 4 whole wheat tortillas
- Salsa and guacamole (optional)
- Salt and pepper to taste

NUTRITIONAL VALUES (APPROXIMATE):

- Calories: 300 (per serving)
- Carbohydrates: 55g
- Protein: 10g
- Fat: 5g
- Fiber: 10g
- Sugar: 4g

INSTRUCTIONS:

1. In a pan, add black beans and mixed veggies. Cook till heated thoroughly.
2. Warm the whole wheat tortillas.
3. Spoon the bean and veggie mixture over each tortilla, add salsa and guacamole if preferred, wrap up, and serve.

RED BEANS WITH RICE

- Prep Time: 10 minutes
- Cooking Time: 30 minutes
- Servings: 4

INGREDIENTS:

- 1 cup long-grain brown rice
- 1 can (15 Oz) red beans, drained and rinsed
- 1/2 cup bell pepper, chopped
- 1/2 cup onion, chopped
- 1 teaspoon Cajun seasoning
- Salt and pepper to taste

NUTRITIONAL VALUES (APPROXIMATE):

- Calories: 250 (per serving)
- Carbohydrates: 52g
- Protein: 7g
- Fat: 1g
- Fiber: 6g
- Sugar: 3g

INSTRUCTIONS:

1. Cook brown rice according per package directions.
2. In a pan, sauté bell pepper and onion until tender.
3. Add red beans, Cajun spice, salt, and pepper. Cook till heated thoroughly.
4. Serve the red beans over cooked brown rice.

WHITE BEANS WITH SPINACH AND PAN-ROASTED

- Prep Time: 15 minutes
- Cooking Time: 20 minutes
- Servings: 4

INGREDIENTS:

- 2 cans (15 Oz each) white beans, drained and rinsed
- 2 cups fresh spinach
- 1 cup cherry tomatoes
- 2 cloves garlic, minced
- 2 tablespoons olive oil
- Salt and pepper to taste

NUTRITIONAL VALUES (APPROXIMATE):

- Calories: 200 (per serving)
- Carbohydrates: 30g
- Protein: 9g
- Fat: 7g
- Fiber: 8g
- Sugar: 2g

INSTRUCTIONS:

1. In a pan, heat olive oil and sauté minced garlic.
2. Add cherry tomatoes and heat until they blister.
3. Add white beans and spinach, and simmer until the spinach wilts.
4. Season with salt and pepper.

TOFU WITH BRUSSELS SPROUTS

- Prep Time: 10 minutes
- Cooking Time: 15 minutes
- Servings: 4

INGREDIENTS:

- 1 block of firm tofu, cubed 2 cups Brussels sprouts, half
- 2 tablespoons soy sauce (low-sodium)
- 1 tablespoon olive oil
- Salt and pepper to taste

NUTRITIONAL VALUES
(APPROXIMATE):

- Calories: 180 (per serving)
- Carbohydrates: 10g
- Protein: 15g
- Fat: 10g
- Fiber: 5g
- Sugar: 2g

INSTRUCTIONS:

1. Heat olive oil in a skillet.
2. Add tofu and Brussels sprouts, sauté until just browned.
3. Pour in soy sauce and simmer for a few more minutes until cooked through.

TOFU WITH PEAS

- Prep Time: 10 minutes
- Cooking Time: 15 minutes
- Servings: 4

INGREDIENTS:

- 1 brick of firm tofu, cubed
- 1 cup peas (fresh or frozen)
- 1/4 cup vegetable broth
- 2 tablespoons soy sauce (low-sodium)
- 1 tablespoon sesame oil
- Salt and pepper to taste

NUTRITIONAL VALUES
(APPROXIMATE):

- Calories: 190 (per serving)
- Carbohydrates: 8g
- Protein: 15g
- Fat: 11g
- Fiber: 2g
- Sugar: 2g

INSTRUCTIONS:

1. In a pan, sauté cubed tofu until gently browned.
2. Add peas, vegetable broth, soy sauce, sesame oil, salt, and pepper.
3. Cook until peas are soft and tofu is cooked through.

BROWN RICE PILAF

🦪 **Prep Time: 10 minutes**

🦪 **Cooking Time: 30 minutes**

🦪 **Servings: 4**

INGREDIENTS:

- 1 cup brown rice
- 2 cups vegetable broth
- 1/2 cup mixed veggies (e.g., carrots, peas, corn)
- 2 cloves garlic, minced
- 2 tablespoons olive oil
- Salt and pepper to taste

NUTRITIONAL VALUES (APPROXIMATE):

- Calories: 180 (per serving)
- Carbohydrates: 35g
- Protein: 4g
- Fat: 3.5g
- Fiber: 3g
- Sugar: 2g

INSTRUCTIONS:

1. In a saucepan, heat olive oil and sauté minced garlic.
2. Add brown rice and mixed veggies. Cook for a few minutes.
3. Pour in vegetable broth, salt, and pepper. Simmer for around 30 minutes or until the rice is cooked and the liquid is absorbed.

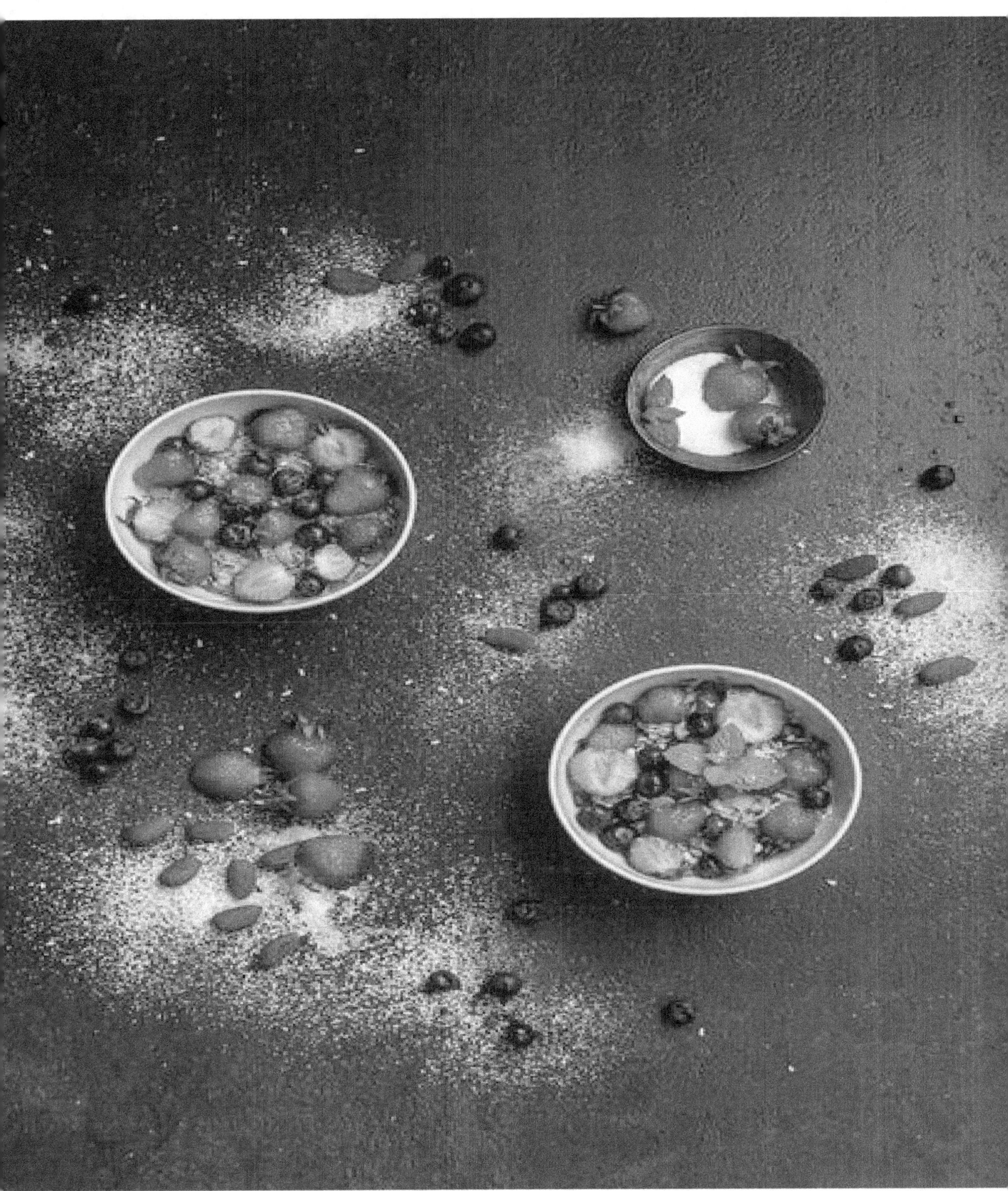

NORI WRAPS WITH FRESH VEGETABLES AND QUINOA

- Prep Time: 20 minutes
- Servings: 4

INGREDIENTS:

- 4 sheets of nori seaweed
- 1 cup cooked quinoa
- Assorted fresh veggies (e.g., cucumber, carrot, bell pepper)
- Soy sauce or tamari for dipping

NUTRITIONAL VALUES (APPROXIMATE):

- Calories: 150 (per serving)
- Carbohydrates: 30g
- Protein: 5g
- Fat: 1g
- Fiber: 5g
- Sugar: 2g

INSTRUCTIONS:

1. Lay down a sheet of nori seaweed.
2. Spread a layer of cooked quinoa on the nori.
3. Add julienned fresh veggies.
4. Roll up the nori and slice into bite-sized pieces. Serve with soy sauce or tamari for dipping.

KALE WRAPS WITH CHILI, GARLIC, CUCUMBER, CORIANDER, AND GREEN BEANS

- Prep Time: 15 minutes
- Servings: 4

INGREDIENTS:

- Large kale leaves, destemmed
- Sliced cucumber
- Green beans, blanched
- Chopped fresh coriander
- Sliced chili pepper
- Minced garlic

NUTRITIONAL VALUES (APPROXIMATE):

- Calories: 80 (per serving)

- Carbohydrates: 15g
- Protein: 4g
- Fat: 1g
- Fiber: 4g
- Sugar: 2g

1. Lay out kale leaves.
2. Fill with cucumber, green beans, coriander, chili, and garlic.
3. Roll up the kale leaves and fasten with toothpicks.

CABBAGE WRAPS WITH AVOCADO, ASPARAGUS, PECAN NUTS, AND STRAWBERRIES

- Prep Time: 20 minutes
- Servings: 4

INGREDIENTS:

- Large cabbage leaves
- Sliced avocado
- Blanched asparagus spears
- Pecan nuts
- Sliced strawberries

NUTRITIONAL VALUES (APPROXIMATE):

- Calories: 120 (per serving)
- Carbohydrates: 12g
- Protein: 3g
- Fat: 7g
- Fiber: 4g
- Sugar: 4g

INSTRUCTIONS:

1. Lay out cabbage leaves.
2. Fill with avocado, asparagus, pecan nuts, and strawberries.
3. Roll up the cabbage leaves and fasten with toothpicks.

BAKED EGGS IN AVOCADO

- Prep Time: 10 minutes
- Cooking Time: 15 minutes
- Servings: 4

INGREDIENTS:

- 4 avocados, halved and pitted
- 4 eggs
- Salt and pepper to taste
- Optional toppings: salsa, chopped herbs, or cheese

- Calories: 180 (per serving)
- Carbohydrates: 7g
- Protein: 7g
- Fat: 15g
- Fiber: 5g
- Sugar: 1g

INSTRUCTIONS:

1. Preheat the oven to 375°F (190°C).
2. Scoop off a little bit of each avocado half to make place for the egg.
3. Crack an egg into each avocado half, then season with salt and pepper.
4. Bake for around 15 minutes or until the egg is cooked to your preferred degree.
5. Add optional toppings, if desired.

TOMATO AND GUACA SALAD

- Prep Time: 10 minutes
- Servings: 4

INGREDIENTS:

- 2 cups cherry tomatoes, halved 1 avocado, diced 1/2 red onion, finely chopped 1/4 cup cilantro, chopped Juice of 2 limes
- Salt and pepper to taste

NUTRITIONAL VALUES (APPROXIMATE):

- Calories: 100 (per serving)
- Carbohydrates: 9g
- Protein: 2g
- Fat: 7g
- Fiber: 4g
- Sugar: 3g

INSTRUCTIONS:

- In a bowl, add cherry tomatoes, avocado, red onion, and cilantro.
- Drizzle with lime juice and season with salt and pepper.

THREE BEAN AND SCALLION SALAD

- Prep Time: 15 minutes
- Servings: 4

INGREDIENTS:

- 1 can (15 oz) black beans, drained and rinsed
- 1 can (15 oz) kidney beans, drained and rinsed
- 1 can (15 oz) garbanzo beans, drained and rinsed
- 4 onions, chopped 2 tablespoons olive oil
- 2 teaspoons red wine vinegar
- Salt and pepper to taste

NUTRITIONAL VALUES (APPROXIMATE):

- Calories: 220 (per serving)
- Carbohydrates: 36g
- Protein: 10g
- Fat: 6g
- Fiber: 12g
- Sugar: 2g

INSTRUCTIONS:

- In a bowl, add black beans, kidney beans, garbanzo beans, and onions.
- Drizzle with olive oil and red wine vinegar. Season with salt and pepper.

CHERRY TOMATO SALAD

- Prep Time: 10 minutes
- Servings: 4

INGREDIENTS:

- 2 cups cherry tomatoes, halved
- 1/2 cup fresh mozzarella balls, halved
- 1/4 cup fresh basil leaves
- 2 tablespoons balsamic vinegar
- 1 tablespoon olive oil
- Salt and pepper to taste

NUTRITIONAL VALUES (APPROXIMATE):

- Calories: 160 (per serving)
- Carbohydrates: 7g
- Protein: 6g
- Fat: 11g
- Fiber: 1g
- Sugar: 4g

INSTRUCTIONS:

- In a bowl, add cherry tomatoes, mozzarella balls, and fresh basil leaves.
- Drizzle with balsamic vinegar and olive oil. Season with salt and pepper.

ASIAN CUCUMBER SALAD

- Prep Time: 10 minutes
- Servings: 4

INGREDIENTS:

- 2 cucumbers, thinly sliced
- 2 tablespoons rice vinegar
- 1 tablespoon soy sauce (low-sodium)
- 1 tablespoon sesame oil
- 1 teaspoon honey or agave syrup
- Sesame seeds (for garnish)

NUTRITIONAL VALUES (APPROXIMATE):

- Calories: 60 (per serving)
- Carbohydrates: 8g
- Protein: 2g
- Fat: 2g
- Fiber: 2g
- Sugar: 4g

INSTRUCTIONS:

1. In a bowl, mix cucumber slices.
2. In a separate bowl, mix together rice vinegar, soy sauce, sesame oil, and honey.
3. Pour the dressing over the cucumbers, stir to coat, and sprinkle with sesame seeds.

SCALLOP CAESAR SALAD

- Prep Time: 15 minutes
- Servings: 4

INGREDIENTS:

- 1 pound scallops
- Romaine lettuce, chopped Caesar dressing
- Grated Parmesan cheese
- Croutons

NUTRITIONAL VALUES (APPROXIMATE):

- Calories: 250 (per serving)
- Carbohydrates: 7g
- Protein: 20g
- Fat: 15g
- Fiber: 2g
- Sugar: 1g

INSTRUCTIONS:

1. Season scallops with salt and pepper and sear in a hot pan until done.
2. Toss romaine lettuce with Caesar dressing.

3. Top with cooked scallops, grated Parmesan cheese, and croutons.

CALIFORNIA WRAPS

Prep Time: 15 minutes

Servings: 4

INGREDIENTS:

- Large lettuce leaves (e.g., iceberg or butter head)
- Sliced avocado
- Sliced turkey or chicken breast
- Sliced cheese (e.g., Swiss or cheddar)
- Sliced tomatoes
- Mayonnaise or mustard (optional)

NUTRITIONAL VALUES (APPROXIMATE):

- Calories: 250 (per serving)
- Carbohydrates: 8g
- Protein: 18g
- Fat: 15g
- Fiber: 4g
- Sugar: 2g

INSTRUCTIONS:

1. Lay out big lettuce leaves.
2. Fill with avocado, turkey or chicken, cheese, and tomatoes.
3. Add mayonnaise or mustard if desired.
4. Roll up the lettuce leaves to make wraps.

CUCUMBER SALAD

Prep Time: 10 minutes

Servings: 4

INGREDIENTS:

- 2 cucumbers, cut 1/2 red onion, finely sliced
- 1/4 cup white wine vinegar
- 2 tablespoons olive oil
- 1 tablespoon fresh dill, chopped
- Salt and pepper to taste

NUTRITIONAL VALUES (APPROXIMATE):

- Calories: 70 (per serving)
- Carbohydrates: 6g
- Protein: 1g
- Fat: 5g
- Fiber: 2g

- Sugar: 3g

INSTRUCTIONS:

1. In a bowl, add cucumber slices and red onion.

2. In a separate dish, mix together white wine vinegar, olive oil, fresh dill, salt, and pepper.

3. Pour the dressing over the cucumbers and onions and toss to mix.

PERFECT QUINOA SALAD

- Prep Time: 15 minutes
- Servings: 4

INGREDIENTS:

- 2 cups cooked quinoa
- Diced cucumber
- Cherry tomatoes, halved
- Diced red bell pepper
- Chopped fresh parsley
- Lemon vinaigrette dressing

NUTRITIONAL VALUES (APPROXIMATE):

- Calories: 180 (per serving)
- Carbohydrates: 30g
- Protein: 5g
- Fat: 4g
- Fiber: 4g
- Sugar: 3g

INSTRUCTIONS:

1. In a bowl, add cooked quinoa, cucumber, cherry tomatoes, red bell pepper, and parsley.
2. Drizzle with lemon vinaigrette dressing and stir to mix.

CUCUMBER, TOMATO, AND AVOCADO SALAD

- Prep Time: 10 minutes
- Servings: 4

INGREDIENTS:

- 2 cucumbers, sliced 2 cups cherry tomatoes, halved 2 avocados, diced 1/4 cup red onion, coarsely chopped Fresh basil leaves

- Balsamic vinaigrette dressing

NUTRITIONAL VALUES (APPROXIMATE):

- Calories: 180 (per serving)
- Carbohydrates: 15g
- Protein: 3g
- Fat: 15g
- Fiber: 7g

- Sugar: 5g

INSTRUCTIONS:

1. In a bowl, add cucumbers, cherry tomatoes, avocados, red onion, and fresh basil leaves.
2. Drizzle with balsamic vinaigrette dressing and stir to mix.

THREE BEAN AND BASIL SALAD

Prep Time: 15 minutes

Servings: 4

INGREDIENTS:

- 1 can (15 oz) kidney beans, drained and rinsed
- 1 can (15 oz) black beans, drained and rinsed
- 1 can (15 oz) garbanzo beans, drained and rinsed
- Fresh basil leaves, chopped 2 cloves garlic, minced 2 tablespoons olive oil
- Salt and pepper to taste

NUTRITIONAL VALUES (APPROXIMATE):

- Calories: 200 (per serving)
- Carbohydrates: 30g
- Protein: 10g
- Fat: 6g
- Fiber: 10g
- Sugar: 3g

INSTRUCTIONS:

1. In a bowl, add kidney beans, black beans, garbanzo beans, basil leaves, and chopped garlic.
2. Drizzle with olive oil, then season with salt and pepper.

TABBOULEH - ARABIAN SALAD

- 🦪 **Prep Time:** 20 minutes
- 🦪 **Servings:** 4

INGREDIENTS:

- 1 cup bulgur wheat
- 2 cups water
- 1 cup fresh parsley, chopped
- 1/2 cup fresh mint leaves, chopped 2 tomatoes, diced 1 cucumber, diced
- Juice of 2 lemons
- Olive oil, to taste
- Salt and pepper to taste

NUTRITIONAL VALUES (APPROXIMATE):

- Calories: 160 (per serving)
- Carbohydrates: 34g
- Protein: 4g
- Fat: 1g
- Fiber: 9g
- Sugar: 2g

INSTRUCTIONS:

1. Combine bulgur wheat and water in a bowl, let rest for approximately 20 minutes until the wheat is mushy and has absorbed the water.
2. Fluff the wheat with a fork and let it cool.
3. In a separate bowl, add bulgur, fresh parsley, fresh mint, tomatoes, cucumber, lemon juice, olive oil, salt, and pepper. Toss to blend.

BACON-BROCCOLI SALAD

- 🦪 **Prep Time:** 15 minutes
- 🦪 **Servings:** 4

INGREDIENTS:

- 2 cups broccoli florets
- 1/2 cup crumbled bacon 1/4 cup red onion, coarsely chopped
- 1/4 cup mayonnaise
- 2 teaspoons apple cider vinegar
- 1 tablespoon honey
- Salt and pepper to taste

NUTRITIONAL VALUES (APPROXIMATE):

- Calories: 220 (per serving)
- Carbohydrates: 10g

- Protein: 5g
- Fat: 17g
- Fiber: 2g
- Sugar: 7g

INSTRUCTIONS:

1. In a large bowl, mix broccoli florets, crumbled bacon, and red onion.
2. In a separate dish, mix together mayonnaise, apple cider vinegar, honey, salt, and pepper.
3. Pour the dressing over the broccoli mixture and toss to coat.

BARLEY VEGGIE SALAD

Prep Time: 15 minutes

Servings: 4

INGREDIENTS:

- 1 cup boiled barley
- Diced bell peppers (different hues)
- Diced zucchini
- Sliced black olives
- Crumbled feta cheese
- Olive oil and lemon juice dressing
- Fresh oregano leaves

NUTRITIONAL VALUES (APPROXIMATE):

- Calories: 220 (per serving)
- Carbohydrates: 30g
- Protein: 6g
- Fat: 9g
- Fiber: 6g
- Sugar: 4g

INSTRUCTIONS:

1. In a bowl, add cooked barley, chopped bell peppers, diced zucchini, black olives, and crumbled feta cheese.
2. Drizzle with olive oil and lemon juice dressing, then top with fresh oregano leaves.

CHOPPED VEGGIE SALAD

Prep Time: 15 minutes

Servings: 4

INGREDIENTS:

- Diced cucumber

- Diced red bell pepper

- Cherry tomatoes, halved

- Sliced red onion

- Chopped fresh parsley

- Red wine vinaigrette dressing

- Calories: 70 (per serving)

- Carbohydrates: 15g

- Protein: 2g

- Fat: 1g

- Fiber: 3g

- Sugar: 6g

INSTRUCTIONS:

1. In a bowl, add chopped cucumber, diced red bell pepper, cherry tomatoes, sliced red onion, and fresh parsley.

2. Drizzle with red wine vinaigrette dressing and toss to mix.

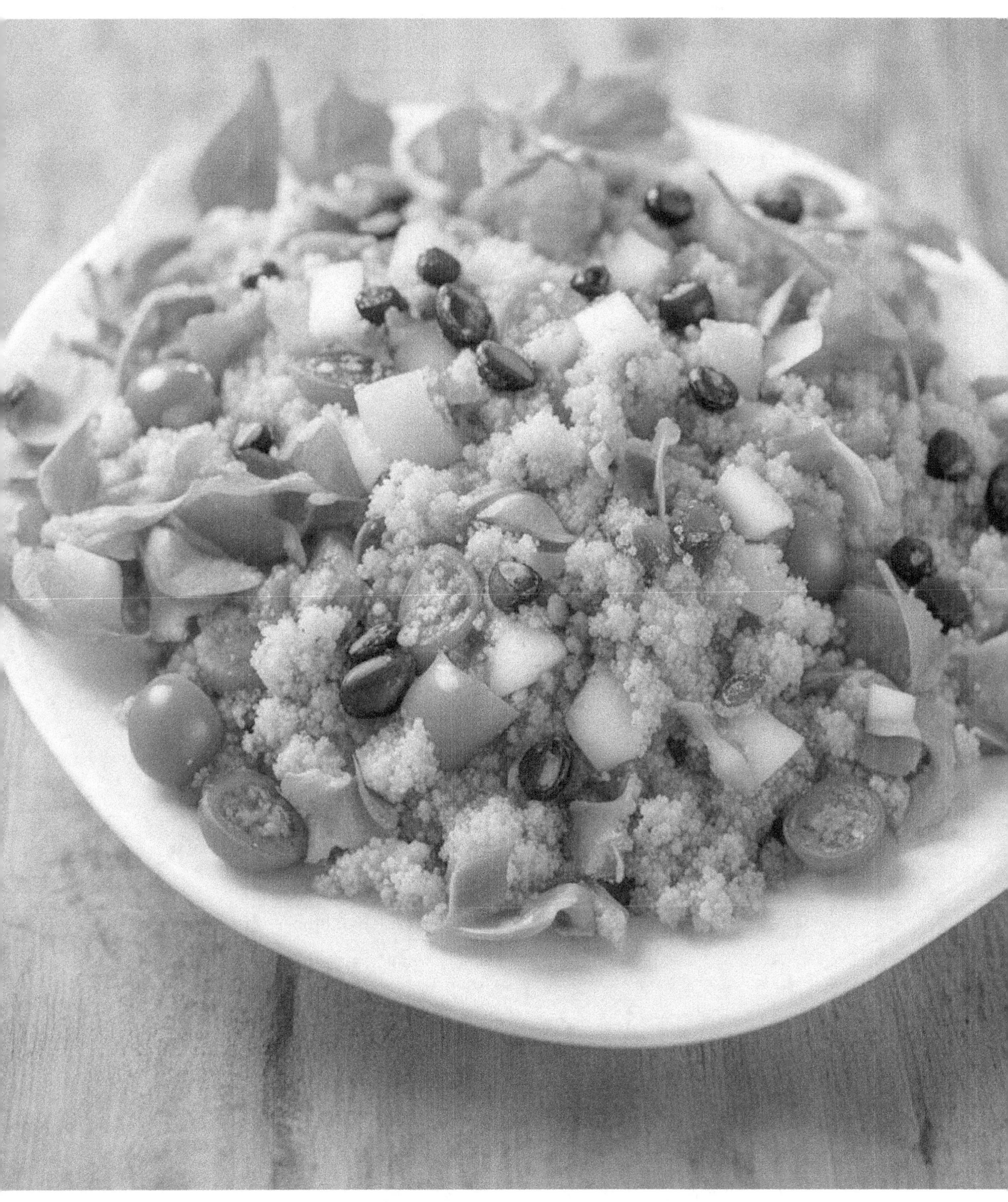

CARROT SOUP WITH TEMPEH

- Prep Time: 15 minutes
- Cooking Time: 30 minutes
- Servings: 4

INGREDIENTS:

- 1 pound carrots, peeled and chopped 8 ounces' tempeh, cubed 1 onion, chopped 2 cloves garlic, minced 4 cups vegetable broth
- 1 teaspoon ginger, grated
- Salt and pepper to taste

NUTRITIONAL VALUES (APPROXIMATE):

- Calories: 200 (per serving)
- Carbohydrates: 20g
- Protein: 14g
- Fat: 8g
- Fiber: 6g
- Sugar: 7g

INSTRUCTIONS:

1. In a large saucepan, sauté onions and garlic until tender.
2. Add carrots, tempeh, ginger, and vegetable broth.
3. Simmer until the carrots are soft.
4. Blend the soup till smooth. Season with salt and pepper.

GINGER, MUSHROOM, AND CAULIFLOWER

- Prep Time: 10 minutes
- Cooking Time: 20 minutes
- Servings: 4

INGREDIENTS:

- 1 head of cauliflower, chopped 8 ounces' mushrooms, sliced 1 onion, chopped 2 cloves garlic, minced 4 cups vegetable broth 1 tablespoon fresh ginger, grated Salt & pepper to taste

NUTRITIONAL VALUES (APPROXIMATE):

- Calories: 120 (per serving)
- Carbohydrates: 20g
- Protein: 7g
- Fat: 2g

- Fiber: 6g
- Sugar: 7g

INSTRUCTIONS:

- In a large saucepan, sauté onions and garlic until tender.

- Add cauliflower, mushrooms, ginger, and vegetable broth.
- Simmer until the veggies are soft.
- Blend the soup till smooth. Season with salt and pepper.

CHICKPEA SOUP

- Prep Time: 15 minutes
- Cooking Time: 25 minutes
- Servings: 4

INGREDIENTS:

- 2 cans (15 oz each) chickpeas, drained and rinsed
- 1 onion, chopped 2 cloves garlic, minced
- 4 cups vegetable broth
- 1 teaspoon cumin
- 1/2 teaspoon paprika
- Salt and pepper to taste

NUTRITIONAL VALUES (APPROXIMATE):

- Calories: 180 (per serving)
- Carbohydrates: 30g
- Protein: 9g
- Fat: 3g
- Fiber: 7g
- Sugar: 6g

INSTRUCTIONS:

1. In a large saucepan, sauté onions and garlic until tender.
2. Add chickpeas, cumin, paprika, and vegetable broth.
3. Simmer for around 20 minutes.
4. Blend a bit of the soup to thicken it. Season with salt and pepper.

PEA AND MINT SOUP

- Prep Time: 10 minutes
- Cooking Time: 20 minutes
- Servings: 4

INGREDIENTS:

- 2 cups frozen peas
- 1 onion, chopped

- 2 cloves garlic, minced
- 4 cups vegetable broth
- 1/4 cup fresh mint leaves
- Salt and pepper to taste

NUTRITIONAL VALUES (APPROXIMATE):

- Calories: 100 (per serving)
- Carbohydrates: 18g
- Protein: 4g
- Fat: 1g

- Fiber: 6g
- Sugar: 6g

INSTRUCTIONS:

1. In a large saucepan, sauté onions and garlic until tender.
2. Add frozen peas, vegetable broth, and fresh mint leaves.
3. Simmer for around 15 minutes.
4. Blend the soup till smooth. Season with salt and pepper.

LENTIL AND EGGPLANT STEW

- Prep Time: 15 minutes
- Cooking Time: 30 minutes
- Servings: 4

INGREDIENTS:

- 1 cup brown lentils, rinsed 1 eggplant, diced 1 onion, chopped 2 cloves garlic, minced 4 cups vegetable broth
- 1 teaspoon cumin
- Salt and pepper to taste

NUTRITIONAL VALUES (APPROXIMATE):

- Calories: 220 (per serving)
- Carbohydrates: 38g
- Protein: 11g
- Fat: 2g
- Fiber: 12g
- Sugar: 6g

INSTRUCTIONS:

1. In a large saucepan, sauté onions and garlic until tender.
2. Add lentils, eggplant, cumin, and vegetable broth.
3. Simmer until lentils and eggplant are soft. Season with salt and pepper.

KALE CAULIFLOWER SOUP

- Prep Time: 15 minutes
- Cooking Time: 25 minutes
- Servings: 4

INGREDIENTS:

- 1 bunch of kale, chopped 1 small head of cauliflower, chopped 1 onion, chopped 2 cloves garlic, minced 4 cups vegetable broth
- 1/2 teaspoon nutmeg
- Salt and pepper to taste

NUTRITIONAL VALUES (APPROXIMATE):

- Calories: 120 (per serving)
- Carbohydrates: 26g
- Protein: 7g
- Fat: 1g
- Fiber: 7g
- Sugar: 4g

INSTRUCTIONS:

1. In a large saucepan, sauté onions and garlic until tender.
2. Add kale, cauliflower, nutmeg, and vegetable broth.
3. Simmer until veggies are soft. Season with salt and pepper.

HEALTHY BROCCOLI ASPARAGUS SOUP

- Prep Time: 10 minutes
- Cooking Time: 20 minutes
- Servings: 4

INGREDIENTS:

- 2 cups broccoli florets
- 2 cups asparagus spears, chopped 1 onion, chopped 2 cloves garlic, minced
- 4 cups vegetable broth
- 1/4 cup plain Greek yogurt
- Salt and pepper to taste

NUTRITIONAL VALUES (APPROXIMATE):

- Calories: 110 (per serving)
- Carbohydrates: 14g

- Protein: 7g
- Fat: 3g
- Fiber: 5g
- Sugar: 6g

INSTRUCTIONS:

1. In a large saucepan, sauté onions and garlic until tender.
2. Add broccoli, asparagus, and vegetable broth.
3. Simmer until veggies are soft.
4. Blend the soup, then whisk in Greek yogurt. Season with salt and pepper.

CREAMY ASPARAGUS SOUP

- Prep Time: 10 minutes
- Cooking Time: 20 minutes
- Servings: 4

INGREDIENTS:

- 2 cups asparagus spears, chopped 1 potato, peeled and chopped 1 onion, chopped 2 cloves garlic, minced
- 4 cups vegetable broth
- 1/2 cup low-fat milk or milk replacement
- Salt and pepper to taste

NUTRITIONAL VALUES (APPROXIMATE):

- Calories: 120 (per serving)
- Carbohydrates: 20g
- Protein: 4g
- Fat: 2g
- Fiber: 4g
- Sugar: 5g

INSTRUCTIONS:

1. In a large saucepan, sauté onions and garlic until tender.
2. Add asparagus, potato, and vegetable broth.
3. Simmer until veggies are soft.
4. Blend the soup and add in low-fat milk. Season with salt and pepper.

- Prep Time: 10 minutes
- Cooking Time: 20 minutes
- Servings: 4

INGREDIENTS:

- 2 cups broccoli florets
- 1 onion, chopped
- 2 cloves garlic, minced
- 4 cups vegetable broth
- 1/4 cup grated Parmesan cheese
- Salt and pepper to taste

NUTRITIONAL VALUES (APPROXIMATE):

- Calories: 110 (per serving)
- Carbohydrates: 10g
- Protein: 7g
- Fat: 5g
- Fiber: 3g
- Sugar: 4g

INSTRUCTIONS:

1. In a large saucepan, sauté onions and garlic until tender.
2. Add broccoli and vegetable broth.
3. Simmer until broccoli is tender.
4. Blend the soup and add in grated Parmesan cheese. Season with salt and pepper.

GREEN LENTIL SOUP

- Prep Time: 15 minutes
- Cooking Time: 30 minutes
- Servings: 4

INGREDIENTS:

- 1 cup green lentils, rinsed 1 onion, chopped 2 cloves garlic, minced 4 cups vegetable broth
- 1 carrot, diced 1 celery stalk, diced 1/2 teaspoon cumin
- Salt and pepper to taste

NUTRITIONAL VALUES (APPROXIMATE):

- Calories: 180 (per serving)
- Carbohydrates: 30g

- Protein: 12g
- Fat: 1g
- Fiber: 12g
- Sugar: 3g

INSTRUCTIONS:

- In a large saucepan, sauté onions and garlic until tender.
- Add green lentils, vegetable broth, carrot, celery, and cumin.
- Simmer for approximately 25 minutes until lentils are cooked. Season with salt and pepper.

SQUASH SOUP

- Prep Time: 15 minutes
- Cooking Time: 30 minutes
- Servings: 4

INGREDIENTS:

- 1 butternut squash, peeled and chopped
- 1 onion, chopped 2 cloves garlic, minced
- 4 cups vegetable broth
- 1/2 teaspoon nutmeg
- Salt and pepper to taste

NUTRITIONAL VALUES (APPROXIMATE):

- Calories: 130 (per serving)
- Carbohydrates: 30g
- Protein: 2g
- Fat: 1g
- Fiber: 5g
- Sugar: 6g

INSTRUCTIONS:

1. In a large saucepan, sauté onions and garlic until tender.
2. Add butternut squash, vegetable broth, and nutmeg.
3. Simmer until squash is soft.
4. Blend the soup and season with salt and pepper.

ROASTED GARLIC SOUP

- Prep Time: 10 minutes
- Cooking Time: 45 minutes
- Servings: 4

INGREDIENTS:

- 2 bulbs of garlic
- 1 onion, chopped

- 4 cups vegetable broth
- 1/4 cup heavy cream or milk replacement
- Fresh thyme leaves
- Salt and pepper to taste

NUTRITIONAL VALUES (APPROXIMATE):

- Calories: 150 (per serving)
- Carbohydrates: 15g
- Protein: 2g
- Fat: 10g
- Fiber: 2g
- Sugar: 3g

INSTRUCTIONS:

1. Roast the garlic bulbs in the oven until tender, then squeeze out the roasted garlic.
2. In a large saucepan, sauté onions till tender.
3. Add the roasted garlic, vegetable broth, and fresh thyme leaves.
4. Simmer for approximately 20 minutes, then mix the soup. Stir in heavy cream or milk substitute. Season with salt and pepper.

GOLDEN MUSHROOM SOUP

- Prep Time: 15 minutes
- Cooking Time: 30 minutes
- Servings: 4

INGREDIENTS:

- 8 oz mushrooms, sliced 1 onion, chopped 2 cloves garlic, minced
- 4 cups vegetable broth
- 1/2 cup light cream or milk replacement
- 2 tablespoons flour
- Fresh thyme leaves
- Salt and pepper to taste

NUTRITIONAL VALUES (APPROXIMATE):

- Calories: 130 (per serving)
- Carbohydrates: 15g
- Protein: 5g
- Fat: 6g
- Fiber: 3g
- Sugar: 5g

INSTRUCTIONS:

1. In a large saucepan, sauté onions, garlic, and mushrooms until tender.

2. Add flour and simmer for a minute.

3. Pour in veggie broth and boil for around 20 minutes.

4. Stir in light cream or milk replacement, fresh thyme leaves, salt, and pepper.

SUMMER VEGETABLE SOUP

- Prep Time: 15 minutes
- Cooking Time: 25 minutes
- Servings: 4

INGREDIENTS:

- Zucchini, diced Yellow squash, diced Red bell pepper, diced Corn kernels
- Onion, chopped 4 cups vegetable broth
- 1/4 cup fresh basil leaves
- Salt and pepper to taste

NUTRITIONAL VALUES (APPROXIMATE):

- Calories: 100 (per serving)
- Carbohydrates: 22g
- Protein: 3g
- Fat: 1g
- Fiber: 5g
- Sugar: 7g

INSTRUCTIONS:

1. In a large saucepan, sauté onions till tender.

2. Add zucchini, yellow squash, red bell pepper, corn, and vegetable broth.

3. Simmer until veggies are soft. Season with salt and pepper. Garnish with fresh basil leaves.

BEET SOUP

- Prep Time: 15 minutes
- Cooking Time: 30 minutes
- Servings: 4

INGREDIENTS:

- 3 beets, peeled and chopped
- 1 onion, chopped 2 cloves garlic, minced
- 4 cups vegetable broth
- 1/4 cup plain Greek yogurt
- Fresh dill leaves
- Salt and pepper to taste

NUTRITIONAL VALUES (APPROXIMATE):

- Calories: 130 (per serving)

- Carbohydrates: 20g

- Protein: 5g

- Fat: 2g

- Fiber: 6g

- Sugar: 10g

INSTRUCTIONS:

1. In a large saucepan, sauté onions and garlic until tender.

2. Add beets and veggie broth.

3. Simmer until beets are soft. Blend the soup and add in Greek yogurt. Season with salt and pepper. Garnish with fresh dill leaves.

VEGGIE STEW

- Prep Time: 15 minutes
- Cooking Time: 30 minutes
- Servings: 4

INGREDIENTS:

- Assorted veggies (carrots, potatoes, bell peppers, etc.), diced

- 1 onion, chopped 2 cloves garlic, minced 4 cups vegetable broth

- 1 can (15 oz) chopped tomatoes

- 1 teaspoon Italian seasoning

- Salt and pepper to taste

NUTRITIONAL VALUES (APPROXIMATE):

- Calories: 120 (per serving)

- Carbohydrates: 25g

- Protein: 4g

- Fat: 1g

- Fiber: 6g

- Sugar: 6g

INSTRUCTIONS:

1. In a large saucepan, sauté onions and garlic until tender.

2. Add mixed veggies, vegetable broth, diced tomatoes, and Italian seasoning.

3. Simmer until veggies are soft. Season with salt and pepper.

ALMOND & RED BELL PEPPER DIP

- Prep Time: 10 minutes
- Servings: 4

INGREDIENTS:

- 2 red bell peppers, roasted and peeled
- 1/2 cup almonds, toasted
- 2 cloves garlic
- 2 tablespoons olive oil
- 1 tablespoon lemon juice
- Salt and pepper to taste

NUTRITIONAL VALUES (APPROXIMATE):

- Calories: 120 (per serving)
- Carbohydrates: 5g
- Protein: 4g
- Fat: 10g
- Fiber: 2g
- Sugar: 2g

INSTRUCTIONS:

1. In a food processor, mix roasted red bell peppers, toasted almonds, garlic, olive oil, and lemon juice.
2. Blend until smooth. Season with salt and pepper.

SPICY CARROT SOUP

- Prep Time: 10 minutes
- Cooking Time: 25 minutes
- Servings: 4

INGREDIENTS:

- 1 pound carrots, chopped 1 onion, chopped 2 cloves garlic, minced
- 4 cups vegetable broth
- 1/2 teaspoon curry powder
- 1/4 teaspoon cayenne pepper
- Salt and pepper to taste

NUTRITIONAL VALUES (APPROXIMATE):

- Calories: 90 (per serving)
- Carbohydrates: 20g
- Protein: 2g
- Fat: 1g
- Fiber: 5g
- Sugar: 8g

INSTRUCTIONS:

1. In a large saucepan, sauté onions and garlic until tender.

2. Add carrots, vegetable broth, curry powder, and cayenne pepper.

3. Simmer until carrots are soft. Season with salt and pepper.

ZUCCHINI SOUP

- Prep Time: 10 minutes
- Cooking Time: 20 minutes
- Servings: 4

INGREDIENTS:

- 4 zucchinis, sliced 1 onion, chopped 2 cloves garlic, minced
- 4 cups vegetable broth
- 1/4 cup plain Greek yogurt
- Fresh basil leaves
- Salt and pepper to taste

NUTRITIONAL VALUES (APPROXIMATE):

- Calories: 90 (per serving)
- Carbohydrates: 15g
- Protein: 4g
- Fat: 2g
- Fiber: 4g
- Sugar: 7g

INSTRUCTIONS:

1. In a large saucepan, sauté onions and garlic until tender.

2. Add zucchinis and veggie broth.

3. Simmer until zucchinis are soft. Blend the soup and add in Greek yogurt. Season with salt and pepper. Garnish with fresh basil leaves.

CABBAGE SOUP

- Prep Time: 15 minutes
- Cooking Time: 30 minutes
- Servings: 4

INGREDIENTS:

- 1 small head of cabbage, shredded
- 1 onion, chopped 2 cloves garlic, minced
- 4 cups vegetable broth
- 1 can (15 oz) chopped tomatoes
- 1 teaspoon Italian seasoning
- Salt and pepper to taste

- Calories: 80 (per serving)
- Carbohydrates: 20g
- Protein: 3g
- Fat: 1g
- Fiber: 6g
- Sugar: 10g

INSTRUCTIONS:

1. In a large saucepan, sauté onions and garlic until tender.
2. Add shredded cabbage, vegetable broth, chopped tomatoes, and Italian spice.
3. Simmer until the cabbage is soft. Season with salt and pepper.

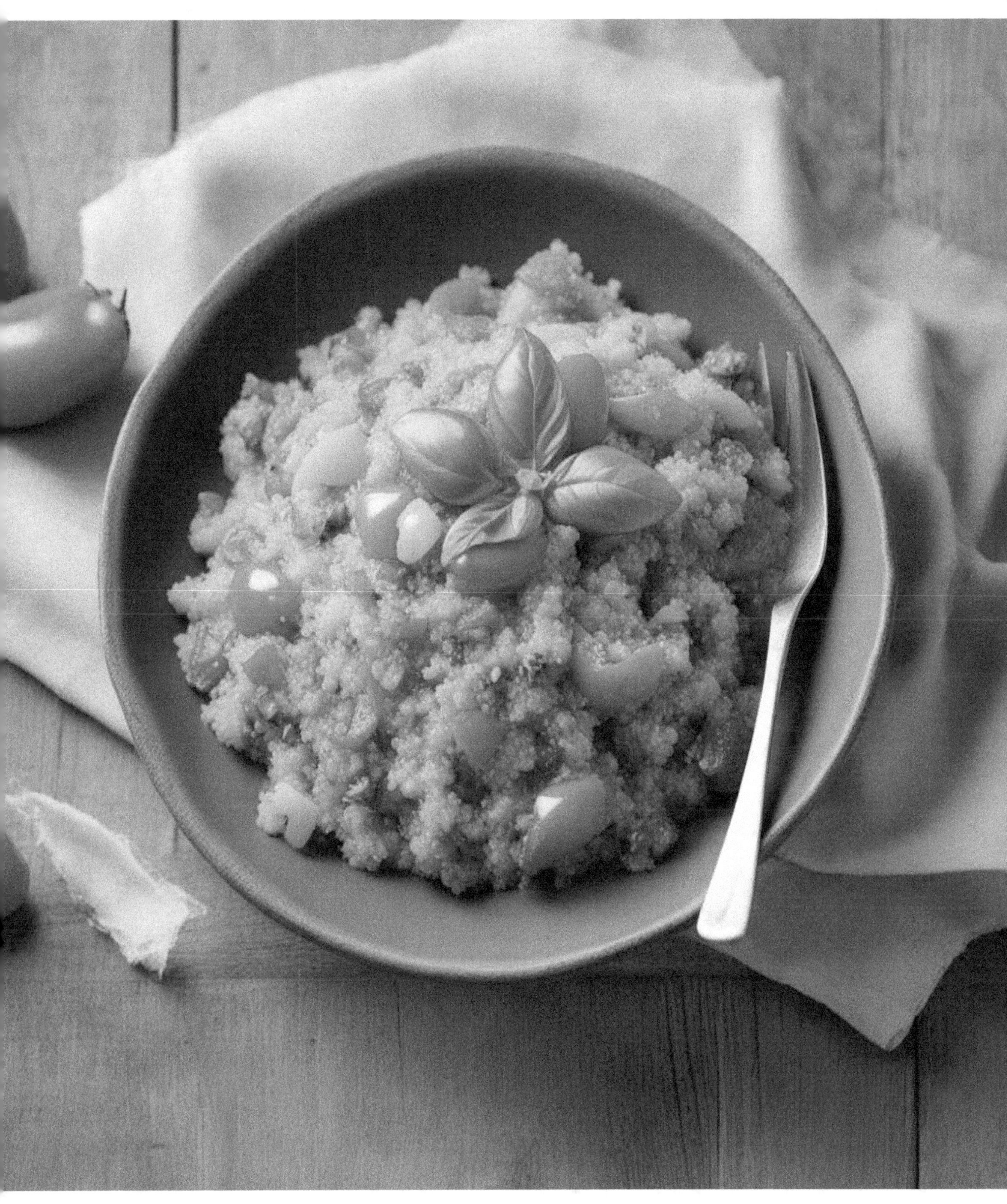

COCONUT MILK PEAR SHAKE

Prep Time: 5 minutes

Servings: 2

INGREDIENTS:

- 2 ripe pears, peeled and cored
- 1 cup coconut milk
- 1 tablespoon honey or maple syrup
- 1/2 teaspoon vanilla extract
- Ice cubes (optional)

NUTRITIONAL VALUES (APPROXIMATE):

- Calories: 180 (per serving)
- Carbohydrates: 30g
- Protein: 2g
- Fat: 7g
- Fiber: 6g
- Sugar: 18g

INSTRUCTIONS:

1. Place pears, coconut milk, honey or maple syrup, and vanilla extract in a blender.
2. Blend until smooth. Add ice cubes if required and mix again.

APPLE, BERRIES, AND KALE SMOOTHIE

Prep Time: 5 minutes

Servings: 2

INGREDIENTS:

- 1 apple, cored and cut
- 1 cup mixed berries (e.g., strawberries, blueberries)
- 1 cup kale leaves, stems removed
- 1 cup water or unsweetened almond milk
- 1 tbsp. chia seeds
- Ice cubes (optional)

NUTRITIONAL VALUES (APPROXIMATE):

- Calories: 120 (per serving)
- Carbohydrates: 25g
- Protein: 3g
- Fat: 2g

- Fiber: 7g
- Sugar: 13g

INSTRUCTIONS:

1. Place apple, mixed berries, kale, water or almond milk, and chia seeds in a blender.
2. Blend until smooth. Add ice cubes if required and mix again.

ORANGE BANANA SMOOTHIE

Prep Time: 5 minutes

Servings: 2

INGREDIENTS:

- 2 ripe bananas
- 2 oranges, peeled and sliced
- 1/2 cup Greek yogurt or yogurt substitute
- 1/2 cup water or orange juice
- Honey or maple syrup (optional, for sweetness)

NUTRITIONAL VALUES (APPROXIMATE):

- Calories: 150 (per serving)
- Carbohydrates: 35g
- Protein: 5g
- Fat: 1g
- Fiber: 5g
- Sugar: 23g

INSTRUCTIONS:

1. Place bananas, oranges, Greek yogurt, water or orange juice, and sugar (if preferred) in a blender.
2. Blend until smooth.

STRAWBERRY APPLE JUICE

Prep Time: 5 minutes

Servings: 2

INGREDIENTS:

- 1 cup strawberries, hulled 2 apples, cored and chopped 1/2 cup water
- 1 tablespoon honey or maple syrup (optional)

NUTRITIONAL VALUES (APPROXIMATE):

- Calories: 90 (per serving)

- Carbohydrates: 22g

- Protein: 1g

- Fat: 1g

- Fiber: 4g

- Sugar: 16g

INSTRUCTIONS:

1. Place strawberries, apples, water, and sweetener (if preferred) in a blender.
2. Blend until smooth.

AUTUMN ENERGIZER JUICE

Prep Time: 5 minutes

Servings: 2

INGREDIENTS:

- 2 carrots, peeled and sliced
- 2 apples, cored and chopped 1/2 lemon, peeled and seeded
- 1-inch slice of ginger
- Ice cubes (optional)

NUTRITIONAL VALUES (APPROXIMATE):

- Calories: 80 (per serving)
- Carbohydrates: 20g
- Protein: 1g
- Fat: 1g
- Fiber: 4g
- Sugar: 13g

INSTRUCTIONS:

1. Place carrots, apples, lemon, and ginger in a juicer.
2. Process the ingredients to produce fresh juice. Add ice cubes if desired.

GREEN SMOOTHIE

Prep Time: 5 minutes

Servings: 2

INGREDIENTS:

- 2 cups spinach
- 1 cucumber, peeled and cut
- 1 banana
- 1 cup water or coconut water

- 1 tablespoon honey or maple syrup (optional)

NUTRITIONAL VALUES (APPROXIMATE):

- Calories: 80 (per serving)
- Carbohydrates: 18g
- Protein: 2g

- Fat: 1g
- Fiber: 4g
- Sugar: 11g

INSTRUCTIONS:

1. Place spinach, cucumber, banana, water or coconut water, and sugar (if preferred) in a blender.
2. Blend until smooth.

WATERMELON CUCUMBER SMOOTHIE

Prep Time: 5 minutes

Servings: 2

INGREDIENTS:

- 2 cups sliced watermelon
- 1 cucumber, peeled and chopped 1/2 lime, juiced Ice cubes (optional)

NUTRITIONAL VALUES (APPROXIMATE):

- Calories: 50 (per serving)
- Carbohydrates: 13g
- Protein: 1g
- Fat: 0g
- Fiber: 2g
- Sugar: 8g

INSTRUCTIONS:

1. Place watermelon, cucumber, and lime juice in a blender.
2. Blend until smooth. Add ice cubes if desired.

LETTUCE AVOCADO SMOOTHIE

Prep Time: 5 minutes

Servings: 2

INGREDIENTS:

- 2 cups lettuce leaves
- 1 ripe avocado
- 1 banana
- 1 cup water or almond milk
- Honey or maple syrup (optional, for sweetness)

NUTRITIONAL VALUES (APPROXIMATE):

- Calories: 160 (per serving)
- Carbohydrates: 16g
- Protein: 2g
- Fat: 10g

- Fiber: 6g
- Sugar: 6g

INSTRUCTIONS:

1. Place lettuce, avocado, banana, water or almond milk, and sugar (if preferred) in a blender.
2. Blend until smooth.

GREEN BERRY SMOOTHIE

Prep Time: 5 minutes

Servings: 2

INGREDIENTS:

- 1 cup mixed berries (e.g., strawberries, blueberries)
- 1 cup spinach
- 1 banana
- 1 cup water or unsweetened almond milk
- 1 tbsp. chia seeds
- Ice cubes (optional)

NUTRITIONAL VALUES (APPROXIMATE):

- Calories: 120 (per serving)
- Carbohydrates: 25g
- Protein: 3g
- Fat: 2g
- Fiber: 7g
- Sugar: 13g

INSTRUCTIONS:

1. Place mixed berries, spinach, banana, water or almond milk, and chia seeds in a blender.
2. Blend until smooth. Add ice cubes if desired.

GREEN DETOX SMOOTHIE

Prep Time: 5 minutes

Servings: 2

INGREDIENTS:

- 1 cup kale leaves, stems removed
- 1 cucumber, peeled and chopped 1 apple, cored and chopped 1/2 lemon, juiced 1 tablespoon honey or maple syrup (optional)

NUTRITIONAL VALUES (APPROXIMATE):

- Calories: 100 (per serving)
- Carbohydrates: 24g
- Protein: 2g
- Fat: 1g
- Fiber: 6g
- Sugar: 15g

1. Place kale, cucumber, apple, lemon juice, and sweetener (if preferred) in a blender.
2. Blend until smooth.

MANGO BANANA SMOOTHIE

 Prep Time: 5 minutes

 Servings: 2

INGREDIENTS:

- 1 ripe mango, peeled and cut
- 2 bananas
- 1/2 cup Greek yogurt or yogurt substitute
- 1/2 cup water or coconut water
- Honey or maple syrup (optional, for sweetness)

NUTRITIONAL VALUES (APPROXIMATE):

- Calories: 150 (per serving)
- Carbohydrates: 35g
- Protein: 4g
- Fat: 2g
- Fiber: 5g
- Sugar: 25g

INSTRUCTIONS:

1. Place mango, bananas, Greek yogurt, water or coconut water, and sweetener (if preferred) in a blender.
2. Blend until smooth.

APPLE BERRY DETOX SMOOTHIE

- Prep Time: 5 minutes
- Servings: 2

INGREDIENTS:

- 1 apple, cored and cut
- 1 cup mixed berries (e.g., strawberries, blueberries)
- 1 cup water or unsweetened almond milk
- 1 tbsp. chia seeds
- Ice cubes (optional)

NUTRITIONAL VALUES (APPROXIMATE):

- Calories: 120 (per serving)
- Carbohydrates: 25g
- Protein: 3g
- Fat: 2g
- Fiber: 7g
- Sugar: 13g

INSTRUCTIONS:

1. Place apple, mixed berries, water or almond milk, and chia seeds in a blender.
2. Blend until smooth. Add ice cubes if desired.

KALE CITRUS BERRY DETOX SMOOTHIE

- Prep Time: 5 minutes
- Servings: 2

INGREDIENTS:

- 1 cup kale leaves, stems removed
- 1 cup mixed berries (e.g., strawberries, blueberries)
- 1 orange, peeled and segmented
- 1 cup water or orange juice
- 1 tablespoon honey or maple syrup (optional)

NUTRITIONAL VALUES (APPROXIMATE):

- Calories: 140 (per serving)
- Carbohydrates: 30g
- Protein: 3g
- Fat: 1g
- Fiber: 6g
- Sugar: 20g

INSTRUCTIONS:

1. Place kale, mixed berries, orange, water or orange juice, and sugar (if preferred) in a blender.

2. Blend until smooth.

CUCUMBER TOXIN FLUSH SMOOTHIE

🌐 Prep Time: 5 minutes

🌐 Servings: 2

INGREDIENTS:

- 1 cucumber, peeled and chopped 1 lemon, juiced 1 tablespoon fresh ginger, grated 1 cup water or coconut water
- Ice cubes (optional)

NUTRITIONAL VALUES (APPROXIMATE):

- Calories: 90 (per serving)
- Carbohydrates: 8g
- Protein: 1g
- Fat: 0g
- Fiber: 2g
- Sugar: 3g

INSTRUCTIONS:

1. Place cucumber, lemon juice, fresh ginger, water or coconut water, and ice cubes (if preferred) in a blender.

2. Blend until smooth.

CANTALOUPE & PAPAYA SMOOTHIE

🌐 Prep Time: 5 minutes

🌐 Servings: 2

INGREDIENTS:

- 1 cup cantaloupe, chopped 1 cup papaya, chopped 1/2 lime, juiced 1/2 cup coconut water
- Honey or maple syrup (optional, for sweetness)

NUTRITIONAL VALUES (APPROXIMATE):

- Calories: 90 (per serving)
- Carbohydrates: 20g
- Protein: 2g
- Fat: 1g
- Fiber: 4g
- Sugar: 15g

INSTRUCTIONS:

1. Place cantaloupe, papaya, lime juice, coconut water, and sugar (if preferred) in a blender.

2. Blend until smooth.

WATERMELON & CANTALOUPE SMOOTHIE

Prep Time: 5 minutes

Servings: 2

INGREDIENTS:

- 1 cup watermelon, diced 1 cup cantaloupe, diced 1/2 lime, juiced Ice cubes (optional)

NUTRITIONAL VALUES (APPROXIMATE):

- Calories: 40 (per serving)
- Carbohydrates: 10g
- Protein: 1g
- Fat: 0g
- Fiber: 2g
- Sugar: 6g

INSTRUCTIONS:

1. Place watermelon, cantaloupe, lime juice, and ice cubes (if preferred) in a blender.

2. Blend until smooth.

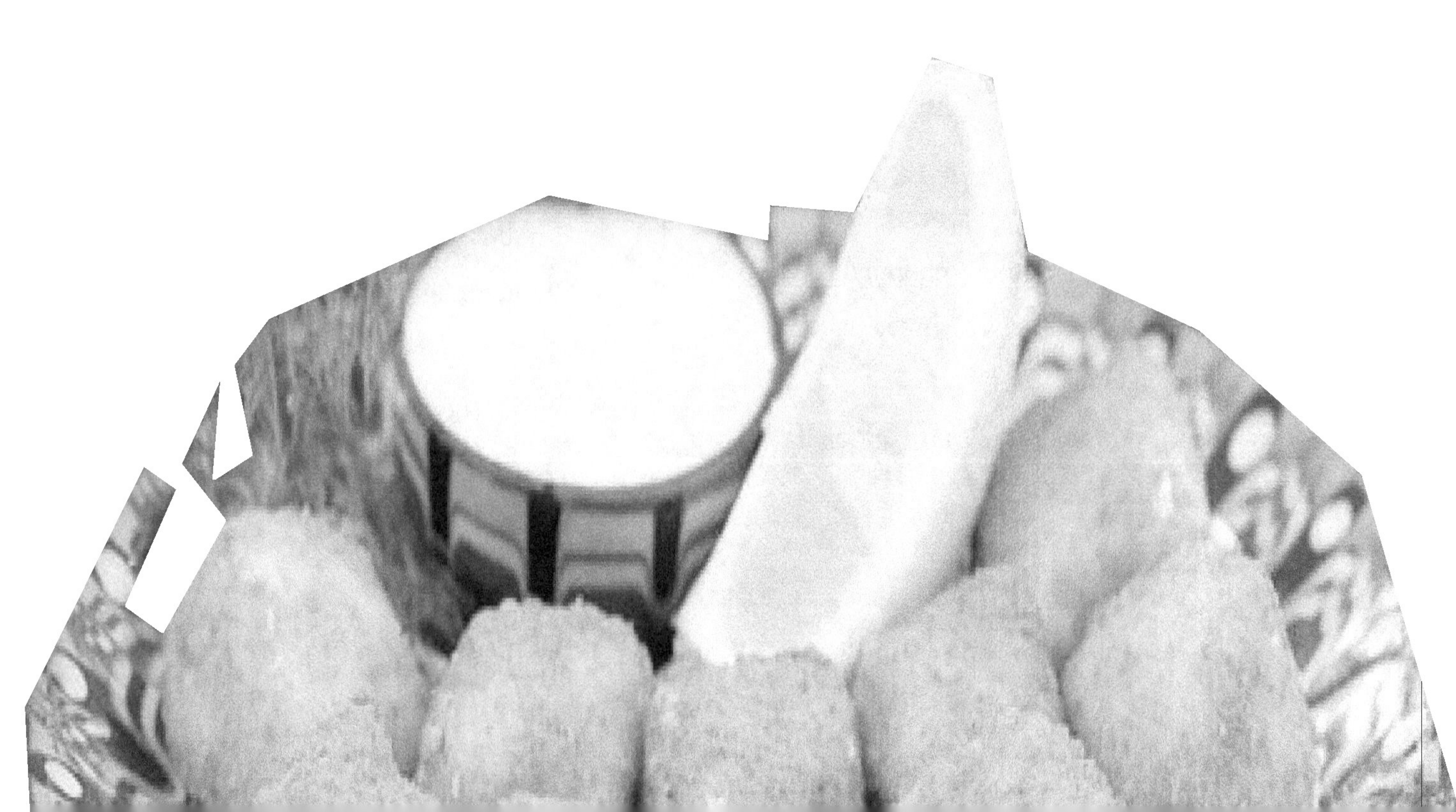

SUNFLOWER SEEDS DRESSING

- Prep Time: 5 minutes
- Servings: 4

INGREDIENTS:

- 1/2 cup sunflower seeds
- 2 tablespoons olive oil
- 1/4 cup water 2 teaspoons lemon juice
- 1 clove garlic
- Salt and pepper to taste

NUTRITIONAL VALUES (APPROXIMATE):

- Calories: 120 (per serving)
- Carbohydrates: 4g
- Protein: 4g
- Fat: 10g
- Fiber: 2g
- Sugar: 1g

INSTRUCTIONS:

1. In a blender, mix sunflower seeds, olive oil, water, lemon juice, garlic, salt, and pepper.
2. Blend until smooth. Adjust consistency with extra water as required.

TOMATO ONION SAUCE

- Prep Time: 10 minutes
- Cooking Time: 15 minutes
- Servings: 4

INGREDIENTS:

- 2 cups chopped tomatoes
- 1 onion, chopped
- 2 cloves garlic, minced
- 1 tablespoon olive oil
- 1/2 teaspoon dried basil
- Salt and pepper to taste

NUTRITIONAL VALUES (APPROXIMATE):

- Calories: 70 (per serving)
- Carbohydrates: 10g
- Protein: 2g
- Fat: 3g

- Fiber: 2g
- Sugar: 5g

INSTRUCTIONS:

1. In a saucepan, heat olive oil and sauté onions and garlic until tender.
2. Add chopped tomatoes, dry basil, salt, and pepper.
3. Simmer for approximately 15 minutes, stirring periodically.

TAMARI & MUSHROOM SAUCE

- Prep Time: 10 minutes
- Cooking Time: 15 minutes
- Servings: 4

INGREDIENTS:

- 1 cup sliced mushrooms
- 1/4 cup tamari sauce (or soy sauce)
- 2 cloves garlic, minced
- 1/2 teaspoon sesame oil
- 1/4 teaspoon ginger, grated

NUTRITIONAL VALUES (APPROXIMATE):

- Calories: 30 (per serving)
- Carbohydrates: 4g
- Protein: 2g
- Fat: 1g
- Fiber: 1g
- Sugar: 1g

INSTRUCTIONS:

1. In a saucepan, add mushrooms, tamari sauce, garlic, sesame oil, and ginger.
2. Simmer for around 15 minutes until the sauce thickens and mushrooms are cooked.

CHUNKY BLACK-BEAN DIP

- Prep Time: 10 minutes
- Servings: 4

INGREDIENTS:

- 1 can (15 oz) black beans, drained and rinsed
- 1/2 cup salsa
- 1/2 cup corn kernels
- 1/4 cup cilantro, chopped
- 1/2 teaspoon cumin
- Salt and pepper to taste

- Calories: 80 (per serving)
- Carbohydrates: 15g
- Protein: 4g
- Fat: 1g
- Fiber: 5g

- Sugar: 1g

INSTRUCTIONS:

1. In a bowl, add black beans, salsa, corn, cilantro, cumin, salt, and pepper.
2. Mash and combine the ingredients to form a thick dip.

ROASTED GARLIC LEMON DIP

Prep Time: 10 minutes

Cooking Time: 25 minutes (for roasting garlic)

Servings: 4

INGREDIENTS:

- 1 entire head of garlic
- 1 tablespoon olive oil
- 1/2 cup Greek yogurt or yogurt substitute
- 1 lemon, juiced
- Salt and pepper to taste

NUTRITIONAL VALUES (APPROXIMATE):

- Calories: 40 (per serving)
- Carbohydrates: 3g
- Protein: 2g
- Fat: 3g
- Fiber: 0g
- Sugar: 1g

INSTRUCTIONS:

1. Preheat your oven to 400°F (200°C).
2. Cut the top off the head of garlic, exposing the cloves.
3. Drizzle with olive oil and cover it in aluminum foil. Roast for approximately 25 minutes until tender and brown.
4. Let the roasted garlic cool, then squeeze out the cloves.
5. In a bowl, mix the roasted garlic, Greek yogurt, lemon juice, salt, and pepper.

SWEET CHILI SAUCE

- Prep Time: 10 minutes
- Cooking Time: 10 minutes
- Servings: 4

INGREDIENTS:

- 1/2 cup rice vinegar
- 1/4 cup water
- 1/4 cup granulated sugar
- 2 cloves garlic, minced
- 2 red chili peppers, coarsely chopped
- 1 tablespoon cornstarch (dissolved in 2 tablespoons of water)

NUTRITIONAL VALUES (APPROXIMATE):

- Calories: 60 (per serving)
- Carbohydrates: 14g
- Protein: 1g
- Fat: 0g
- Fiber: 0g
- Sugar: 11g

INSTRUCTIONS:

1. In a saucepan, add rice vinegar, water, sugar, garlic, and red chili peppers.
2. Bring to a boil, then decrease heat and simmer for approximately 5 minutes.
3. Stir in the cornstarch mixture and boil until the sauce thickens.

TARTAR SAUCE

- Prep Time: 10 minutes
- Servings: 4

INGREDIENTS:

- 1/2 cup mayonnaise or mayonnaise substitute
- 2 tablespoons pickles, finely chopped
- 1 tablespoon capers, chopped
- 1 tablespoon lemon juice
- 1 teaspoon fresh dill, chopped
- Salt and pepper to taste

NUTRITIONAL VALUES (APPROXIMATE):

- Calories: 150 (per serving)
- Carbohydrates: 2g
- Protein: 0g
- Fat: 15g
- Fiber: 0g
- Sugar: 1g

INSTRUCTIONS:

1. In a bowl, add mayonnaise, pickles, capers, lemon juice, fresh dill, salt, and pepper.

BUTTERNUT & TOMATO SPAGHETTI SAUCE

- Prep Time: 15 minutes
- Cooking Time: 30 minutes
- Servings: 4

INGREDIENTS:

- 2 cups butternut squash, chopped
- 1 can (15 oz) chopped tomatoes
- 1 onion, chopped
- 2 cloves garlic, minced
- 1 tablespoon olive oil
- 1 teaspoon Italian seasoning
- Salt and pepper to taste

NUTRITIONAL VALUES (APPROXIMATE):

- Calories: 60 (per serving)
- Carbohydrates: 15g
- Protein: 2g
- Fat: 1g
- Fiber: 4g
- Sugar: 5g

INSTRUCTIONS:

In a saucepan, heat olive oil and sauté onions and garlic until tender.
2. Add butternut squash, diced tomatoes, Italian seasoning, salt, and pepper.
3. Simmer for approximately 30 minutes until the butternut squash is soft.

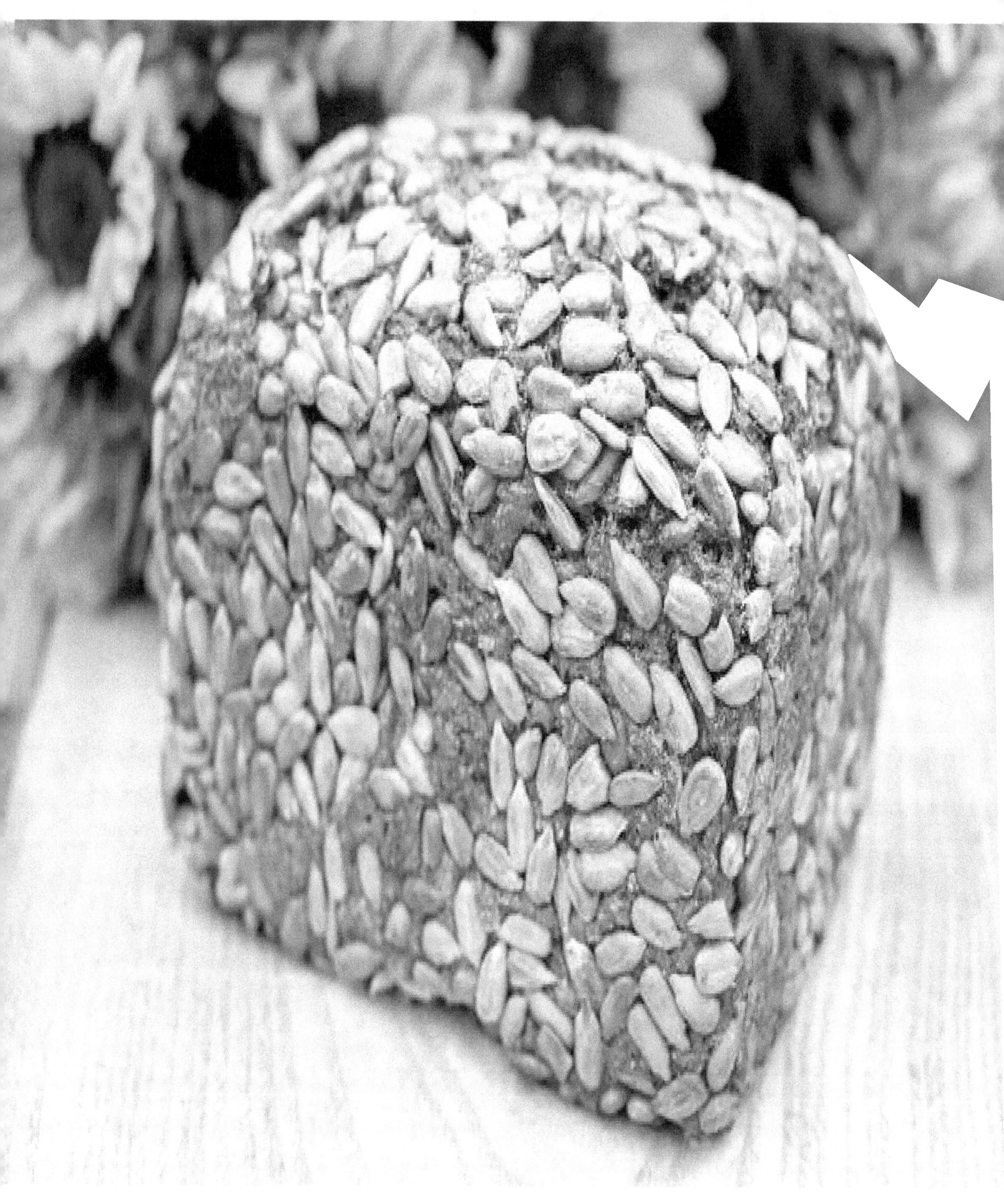

GREEK YOGURT AND BERRIES PARFAIT

- Prep Time: 5 minutes
- Servings: 1

INGREDIENTS:

- 1/2 cup Greek yogurt (low-fat or non-fat)
- 1/2 cup mixed berries (e.g., strawberries, blueberries)
- 1 tablespoon honey or sugar-free sweetener (optional)
- 1 tablespoon chopped nuts (e.g., almonds, walnuts)

NUTRITIONAL VALUES (APPROXIMATE):

- Calories: 180 (per serving)
- Carbohydrates: 20g
- Protein: 15g
- Fat: 6g
- Fiber: 4g
- Sugar: 15g

INSTRUCTIONS:

1. In a serving dish or glass, put Greek yogurt and mixed berries.
2. Drizzle honey or add a sugar-free sweetener if preferred.
3. Sprinkle chopped nuts on top for extra crunch.

CUCUMBER AND HUMMUS SLICES

- Prep Time: 10 minutes
- Servings: 2

INGREDIENTS:

- 1 cucumber, sliced
- 4 tablespoons hummus (low-fat or regular)
- 1 teaspoon fresh dill, chopped Salt and pepper to taste

NUTRITIONAL VALUES (APPROXIMATE):

- Calories: 80 (per serving)
- Carbohydrates: 10g
- Protein: 3g
- Fat: 3g
- Fiber: 3g
- Sugar: 2g

1. Arrange cucumber slices on a platter.

2. Top each cucumber slice with a dab of hummus.

3. Sprinkle with fresh dill, salt, and pepper.

BAKED ZUCCHINI CHIPS

- Prep Time: 15 minutes
- Cooking Time: 25 minutes
- Servings: 2

INGREDIENTS:

- 2 zucchinis, thinly sliced
- 1 tablespoon olive oil
- 1/4 cup grated Parmesan cheese
- 1/2 teaspoon garlic powder
- Salt and pepper to taste

NUTRITIONAL VALUES (APPROXIMATE):

- Calories: 120 (per serving)
- Carbohydrates: 6g
- Protein: 4g
- Fat: 8g
- Fiber: 2g
- Sugar: 3g

INSTRUCTIONS:

1. Preheat your oven to 400°F (200°C) and line a baking sheet with parchment paper.

2. In a bowl, combine zucchini slices with olive oil, Parmesan cheese, garlic powder, salt, and pepper.

3. Arrange the zucchini slices on the baking pan and bake for approximately 20-25 minutes or until they are crispy.

APPLE AND PEANUT BUTTER SLICES

- Prep Time: 5 minutes
- Servings: 1

INGREDIENTS:

- 1 apple, sliced 2 tablespoons natural peanut butter (no added sugar)
- Cinnamon (optional)

NUTRITIONAL VALUES (APPROXIMATE):

- Calories: 250 (per serving)
- Carbohydrates: 25g

- Protein: 7g
- Fat: 15g
- Fiber: 5g
- Sugar: 15g

INSTRUCTIONS:

1. Slice the apple.
2. Spread peanut butter on apple slices.
3. Sprinkle with cinnamon for added taste.

VEGGIE STICKS WITH HUMMUS

- Prep Time: 10 minutes
- Servings: 2

INGREDIENTS:

- Carrot, cucumber, and bell pepper sticks
- 4 tablespoons hummus (low-fat or regular)

NUTRITIONAL VALUES (APPROXIMATE):

- Calories: 60 (per serving)
- Carbohydrates: 10g
- Protein: 2g
- Fat: 2g
- Fiber: 3g
- Sugar: 3g

INSTRUCTIONS:

1. Prepare carrot, cucumber, and bell pepper sticks.
2. Serve with hummus for dipping.

COTTAGE CHEESE AND PINEAPPLE DELIGHT

- Prep Time: 5 minutes
- Servings: 1

INGREDIENTS:

- 1/2 cup low-fat cottage cheese
- 1/2 cup fresh pineapple chunks
- 1 tablespoon chopped fresh mint (optional)

NUTRITIONAL VALUES (APPROXIMATE):

- Calories: 150 (per serving)
- Carbohydrates: 15g
- Protein: 15g
- Fat: 2g
- Fiber: 2g
- Sugar: 10g

INSTRUCTIONS:

1. In a bowl, mix cottage cheese and pineapple chunks.

2. Garnish with chopped fresh mint if preferred.

AVOCADO AND TOMATO SLICES

Prep Time: 5 minutes

Servings: 2

INGREDIENTS:

- 1 avocado, sliced
- 1 tomato, sliced Balsamic vinegar drizzle (optional)
- Salt and pepper to taste

NUTRITIONAL VALUES (APPROXIMATE):

- Calories: 120 (per serving)
- Carbohydrates: 7g
- Protein: 2g
- Fat: 10g
- Fiber: 4g
- Sugar: 2g

INSTRUCTIONS:

1. Arrange avocado and tomato slices on a platter.
2. Drizzle with balsamic vinegar, if preferred.
3. Season with salt and pepper.

WHOLE GRAIN CRACKERS WITH TUNA SALAD

Prep Time: 10 minutes

Servings: 2

INGREDIENTS:

- 1 can (5 oz) tuna, drained
- 2 tablespoons low-fat Greek yogurt
- 1/4 cup sliced celery
- 1/4 cup chopped red onion
- 1 teaspoon Dijon mustard
- Whole grain crackers

NUTRITIONAL VALUES (APPROXIMATE):

- Calories: 150 (per serving)
- Carbohydrates: 10g
- Protein: 15g
- Fat: 5g
- Fiber: 2g
- Sugar: 2g

INSTRUCTIONS:

1. In a bowl, combine tuna, Greek yogurt, celery, red onion, and Dijon mustard.

2. Serve with whole grain crackers.

HARD-BOILED EGGS WITH SPINACH

- Prep Time: 15 minutes
- Cooking Time: 10 minutes
- Servings: 2

INGREDIENTS:

- 4 hard-boiled eggs, sliced 2 cups fresh spinach
- Balsamic vinegar drizzling (optional)
- Salt and pepper to taste

NUTRITIONAL VALUES (APPROXIMATE):

- Calories: 160 (per serving)
- Carbohydrates: 2g
- Protein: 12g
- Fat: 11g
- Fiber: 2g
- Sugar: 0g

INSTRUCTIONS:

1. Arrange hard-boiled egg slices on a bed of fresh spinach.
2. Drizzle with balsamic vinegar if preferred.
3. Season with salt and pepper.

COTTAGE CHEESE AND SLICED PEACHES

- Prep Time: 5 minutes
- Servings: 1

INGREDIENTS:

- 1/2 cup low-fat cottage cheese
- 1 fresh peach, sliced 1 teaspoon honey or sugar-free sweetener (optional)

NUTRITIONAL VALUES (APPROXIMATE):

- Calories: 150 (per serving)
- Carbohydrates: 20g
- Protein: 14g
- Fat: 2g
- Fiber: 2g
- Sugar: 16g

INSTRUCTIONS:

1. In a bowl, add low-fat cottage cheese and sliced peaches.
2. Drizzle with honey or add a sugar-free sweetener if preferred.

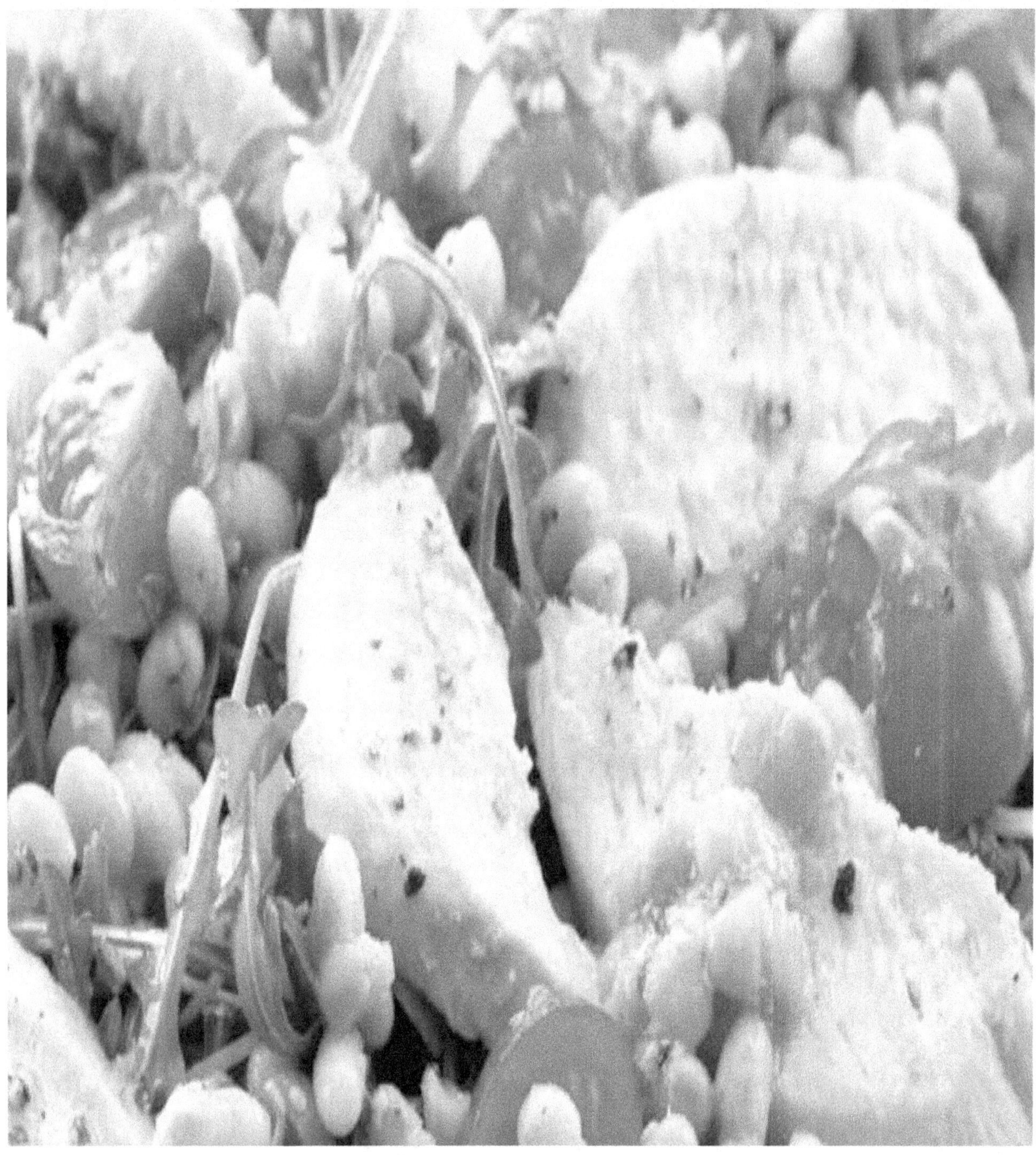

1. What is diabetes?

Answer: Diabetes is a chronic medical illness that affects how your body handles glucose (blood sugar).

2. What are the primary forms of diabetes?

Answer: The primary categories are Type 1, Type 2, and gestational diabetes.

3. What is Type 1 diabetes?

Answer: Type 1 diabetes is an autoimmune disorder in which the body's immune system targets and kills the insulin-producing cells in the pancreas.

4. What is Type 2 diabetes?

Answer: Type 2 diabetes happens when the body gets resistant to insulin or doesn't create enough insulin. It's commonly tied to lifestyle issues.

5. What is gestational diabetes?

Answer: Gestational diabetes develops throughout pregnancy and normally goes away after delivery.

6. What are the common symptoms of diabetes?

Answer: Common symptoms include increased thirst, frequent urination, unexplained weight loss, weariness, and impaired vision.

7. How is diabetes diagnosed?

Answer: Diabetes is commonly diagnosed by blood testing, including fasting blood sugar, oral glucose tolerance test, and HbA1c readings.

8. Can diabetes be prevented?

Answer: Type 1 diabetes cannot be avoided, while Type 2 diabetes may typically be prevented or delayed by lifestyle modifications.

9. How is diabetes treated?

Answer: Treatment may entail lifestyle adjustments, medication, insulin treatment, and monitoring blood sugar levels.

10. What is HbA1c, and why is it crucial for diabetes management?

Answer: HbA1c is a blood test that displays your average blood sugar levels over the last two to three months. It's vital for long-term diabetic control.

11. What are consequences of uncontrolled diabetes?

Answer: Complications may include heart disease, renal disease, neuropathy, retinopathy, and foot difficulties.

12. Can diabetes damage one's mental health?

Answer: Yes, diabetes may contribute to stress, anxiety, and depression owing to the daily management and health issues.

13. How may diet and nutrition assist control diabetes?

Answer: A balanced diet that restricts carbohydrate consumption and focuses on healthy foods may help maintain blood sugar levels.

14. Is exercise helpful for diabetes management?

Answer: Yes, regular physical exercise helps enhance insulin sensitivity and regulate blood sugar levels.

15. Can persons with diabetes consume sweets or sugar?

Answer: Yes, but in moderation. It's crucial to monitor and regulate carbohydrate consumption.

16. What is insulin and when is it used in diabetes treatment?

Answer: Insulin is a hormone used to control blood sugar levels. It's typically recommended for persons with Type 1 diabetes and those with Type 2.

17. Can diabetes be cured?

Answer: There is no treatment for Type 1 diabetes, however Type 2 diabetes may occasionally be treated to the point where it is in remission.

18. Are there any natural therapies for diabetes?

Answer: Some individuals employ alternative treatments; however, they should be reviewed with a healthcare physician.

19. What is hypoglycemia, and how is it treated?

Answer: Hypoglycemia, or low blood sugar, is treated by taking fast-acting carbohydrates, such as glucose tablets or juice.

20. What are the risk factors for acquiring Type 2 diabetes?

Answer: Risk factors include obesity, a sedentary lifestyle, a family history of diabetes, and age.

21. Can diabetes impact pregnancy?

Answer: Yes, gestational diabetes may disrupt pregnancy, but it can frequently be controlled with lifestyle modifications and medication.

22. How frequently should I check my blood sugar levels?

Answer: The frequency of monitoring might vary but is often suggested numerous times a day, particularly if you're using insulin.

23. What is diabetic ketoacidosis (DKA)?

Answer: DKA is a serious complication of diabetes that happens when the body creates excessive quantities of ketones owing to a lack of insulin.

24. Can diabetes lead to cardiac problems?

Answer: Yes, uncontrolled diabetes is a substantial risk factor for heart disease.

25. How can I avoid diabetes complications?

Answer: Proper control of blood sugar, frequent check-ups, a healthy lifestyle, and medication as recommended will help avoid problems.

26. Can diabetes be hereditary?

Answer: Yes, genetics may have a role in the development of diabetes, particularly Type 2 diabetes.

27. Are there support groups for persons with diabetes?

Answer: Yes, many localities offer diabetic support groups, and online networks are accessible as well.

28. Can I consume alcohol if I have diabetes?

Answer: Alcohol may influence blood sugar, thus it should be eaten in moderation and with prudence.

29. Can I travel with diabetes?

Answer: Yes, but it involves organization and preparation, including bringing required supplies and prescriptions.

30. Is it OK to fast on religious holidays if I have diabetes?

Answer: Fasting may be achievable with proper planning and monitoring, but it's vital to check with a healthcare expert.

.

Foods to Eat	Foods to Avoid	Foods to Be Taken Moderately
2. Berries (Blueberries, Strawberries)	2. Processed Meats (Bacon, Sausage)	2. Full-Fat Dairy Products
3. Whole Grains (Quinoa, Oats)	3. Trans Fats (Partially Hydrogenated Oils)	3. White Bread and Pastries
4. Lean Proteins (Chicken, Turkey)	4. Sugary Snacks and Desserts	4. Alcohol (Moderation is key)
5. Fatty Fish (Salmon, Mackerel)	5. Deep-Fried Foods (French Fries)	5. High-Sugar Fruits (Grapes, Watermelon)
6. Nuts and Seeds (Almonds, Chia)	6. Refined Grains (White Rice, White Bread)	6. Processed Foods (Chips, Instant Noodles)
7. Legumes (Beans, Lentils)	7. High-Sodium Foods (Canned Soup)	7. High-Caffeine Beverages (Excessive Coffee)
8. Low-Fat Dairy (Greek Yogurt)	8. Artificial Sweeteners	8. High-Calorie Fast Food (Burgers, Pizza)
9. Avocado	9. Sugary Cereals	9. High-Fat Snacks (Cheese, Butter)
10. Eggs	10. Excess Alcohol Consumption	10. Fruit Juice (High in Added Sugars)
1. Leafy Greens (Spinach, Kale)	1. Sugary Drinks (Soda, Energy Drinks)	1. Red Meat (High in Saturated Fat)

11. Garlic	11. Processed and Red Meats	11. Processed Condiments (Ketchup)
12. Sweet Potatoes	12. High-Fat Dairy (Whole Milk)	12. High-Sugar Condiments (BBQ Sauce)
13. Olive Oil	13. High-Sugar Beverages (Energy Drinks)	13. Highly Processed Snacks (Cookies)
14. Dark Chocolate (Moderation)	14. White Bread	14. Refined Cooking Oils (Vegetable Oil)
15. Citrus Fruits (Oranges, Grapefruits)	15. Highly Processed Snacks (Chips)	15. High-Sodium Sauces (Soy Sauce)
16. Tomatoes	16. High-Sugar Breakfast Cereals	16. High-Caffeine Energy Drinks
17. Onions	17. Fast Food	17. Sugary Alcoholic Drinks (Cocktails)
18. Low-Fat Dairy (Skim Milk)	18. High-Sugar Desserts	18. High-Sugar Sports Drinks
19. Quinoa	19. Artificial Trans Fats (Partially Hydrogenated Oils)	19. Sugary Frozen Desserts (Ice Cream)
20. Green Tea (Moderation)	20. High-Sodium Frozen Meals	20. High-Sugar Salad Dressings

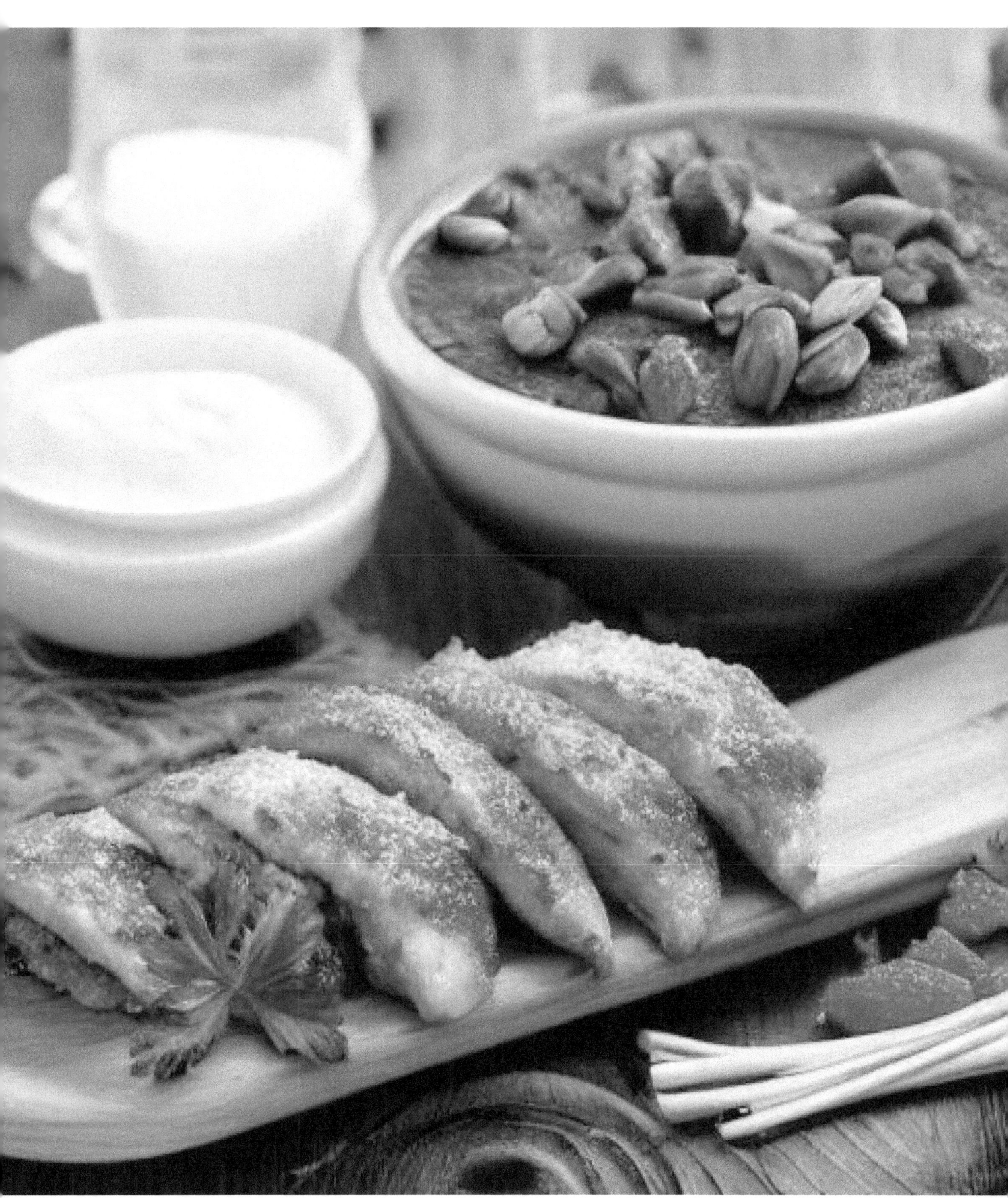

www.ingramcontent.com/pod-product-compliance
Lightning Source LLC
Chambersburg PA
CBHW080823280726
48660CB00019B/3639